Sex Position for Couples

How to use communication, intelligence, energy and fantasy to explore your sexuality. Beginners or not, a guide to improving your sex life.

Sarah Greyhold

Copyright © 2012 Sarah Greyhold
Tutti i diritti riservati.

Codice ISBN:9781708185350

Disclaimer:

Although the author and publisher have made every effort to ensure that the information in this book was correct at press time, the author and publisher do not assume and hereby disclaim any liability to any party for any loss, damage, or disruption caused by errors or omissions, whether such errors or omissions result from negligence, accident, or any other cause.

CONTENTUI

Ch. 1	Importance of Communication in Improving the Sexual Life of the Couple	Pag.4
Ch. 2	Methods to Trigger Sexual Desire in Your Partner	Pag. 13
Ch. 3	Erotic Massage: When to Use It and Bases on How to Practice It	Pag. 23
Ch. 4	Preliminaries: Their Importance, How To Do Them The Best. What She Prefers and What He Prefers.	Pag. 34
Ch. 5	Ten Pleasant Positions for Both	Pag. 51
Ch. 6	Ten Positions Dedicated Mainly To Her, To Give Her Pleasure and Facilitate Orgasm	Pag. 61
Ch. 7	Ten Positions Dedicated Mainly To Him, To Give Him Pleasure and Facilitate Orgasm	Pag.70
Ch. 8	Positions Suitable for Oral Sex Performed On Him	Pag. 80
Ch. 9	Five Positions Suitable for Oral Sex Practiced on Her	Pag. 91
Ch. 10	Five Positions Suitable for Anal Sex in Which She Finds More Pleasure and Less Discomfort	Pag. 100
Ch. 11	Toys: When to Use Them and How	Pag.108

Chapter 1: Importance of Communication in Improving the Sexual Life of the Couple

A happy and successful sexual life requires effective communication from both partners. Cultural backgrounds may hinder this kind of communication but couples must always find ways to get around these obstacles if they want to have a healthy intimate relationship. Communication might vary from one couple to another but it must always meltdown to making sex a fulfilling adventure for both man and woman. We are going to highlight the types of communication before, during and after sex and how they are key to improving a couple's sex life.

Before Sex

Communication before sex is the most important of the three types. The communication or lack of it has the potential to either make or break what you are about to have. This is the time for you to be completely honest about your feelings and other concerns. You should also encourage your partner to speak out their mind so you can know how to handle them. Communication before sex is not just talking, it serves the following purposes as well.

It can be used as foreplay- the words that come out of your mouth should carry a unique taste of sexual desire that sweeps through your partner like a tsunami. The words don't necessarily need to be erotic, the way you say them should have the same effect as erotic ones.

It is a major confidence booster- many people are normally shy during sex especially when they are new to each other. Things that you can't say with your partner or you on top can be said comfortably before sex. Communication reduces tension and makes you feel less vulnerable. Talk about that thing you would like to try before your clothes are off, it will do more good to you than doing it in the course of it when you can't find words to say it. The communication must not always happen face to face, a mere text or phone call can as well work wonders. It will be much easier to revisit the matter when you meet physically. The keyword here is 'creativity'.

Read books or go to the movies- if you think you need more tips to spice up your sex life, you can refer to materials with approved sexual content for that purpose. Maybe you have seen how they do it in a certain movie or book. Ask your partner to accompany you there and see it. Ask if they like it and if it is something the two of you can try on your own.

It helps you to convert memories into new fantasies- if you had done something thrilling sometimes back, you can float the idea to your partner to see if the experience can happen again. It is easier to revisit things that happened in your last sexual encounter than to try things that you have never done before. Your sexual past should be a script for subsequent sex activities. Not only should you pay attention to good experiences, but you should also take note of those that didn't work to avoid repeating them.

It strengthens the bond of intimacy- there is nothing more disturbing than engaging in a sexual act with someone whose mind and emotions are miles away. Communication before sex ensures that both of you are drawn to each other by mutual desire. Let your partner know that he/she is the only thing that matters at that particular moment. Tell them that you want them 100 per cent; their soul, mind, and body. This will draw their attention to that fact and the two of you will be geared towards some mind-blowing sex.

In summary, this is what communication before sex enables both of you to have fulfilling sex:

- It will give you a clue about what you are about to experience.
- It clears the air about things that might be causing you some discomfort, what works and what doesn't work.
- You will be in a better position to satisfy your partner.
- It relieves tension between the two of you.
- It helps both of you identify your most favourite spots to touch during sex.
- It boosts your confidence and eliminates the chances of

you feeling vulnerable during sex.

- It helps both of you to approximate the duration of sex, one that sits well with you as well as your partner.

During Sex

Even though there is a lot of action during the actual sexual process, there also must be plenty of communication with your partner. The communication does not always have to be verbal. It should involve every aspect of you that is mental, physical and emotional communication. Here is how to communicate with your partner during sex and its importance.

Give instructions- ask your partner to touch specific spots briefly and gently as you have sex. Let them know how you feel about their pace, ask them to slow down if they are going fast or increase the pace if you think they are a little slow. The issue of the pace applies to both man and woman, whoever is in control at that particular moment. This helps both of you enjoy sex. Lack of communication and instructions makes it difficult for your partner to figure out how best to handle you. It will also cause you discomfort when your partner is not doing it right.

Talk with your hands most of the time- grab your partner's hand and guide it to that part that gives you the most thrill. Help them massage that clitoris or rub those balls in a pace and intensity that gives you maximum pleasure. Another way of communicating with your hands is not necessarily guiding theirs but just caressing and touching them. Hold your partner's waist and control the thrusts or the rubbing according to the pace of your choice. Guiding their hands to those spots is a way of telling them where to concentrate on as well as the pace that makes you happy.

Combine talking and physical activity- as you do the moaning, try to emphasize it with appropriate actions. Don't just shout 'harder' or 'faster' while behaving like a flag post. Hold your partner's waist and 'harder' with a hard thrust. If you are the one in control, move your body and hands to reinforce your moaning. Your partner will use moaning and sex sounds as a way of giving you positive feedback if you are doing what pleases them.

Facial expressions- it is difficult to tell exactly how your partner is responding to sex but you will an idea from there facial expressions. In most cases, people that ask their partners how they are doing during sex are thought to be underperforming. That is just a fallacy. There is nothing wrong with asking your partner whether they are enjoying it or telling them that you are not enjoying yourself. If your partner makes a move that makes you feel pain or discomfort, you can make a shrieking sound to communicate that to them. Similarly, give heavy moaning sounds whenever they are doing it right.
In summary, communication during sex helps you achieve the

following objectives:

- Ensures that both of you are on the same page, emotionally and mentally, throughout the sex exercise.
- It enables you to learn your partner's body, their weak points and places that cause discomfort.
- It ensures that both of you come out satisfied.
- It ensures that the level of intimacy remains at an all-time high as you have sex.
- It reduces the possibility of one or both partners getting distracted during sex. Constant communication, be it verbal or bodily, draws the attention of both of you.

After Sex

The conversation you have after sex is like a revision of the experience you have just had. This is the point where you analyze sexual performance, yours and that of your partner. You must iron out all the weaknesses and maintain or improve on your strengths before the next sexual encounter. The following are some of the things you should address immediately after that steamy sex.

Start by making the discussion a personal one- tell your partner how you felt during the exercise. Don't be shy to say something you didn't like about the whole thing. Most importantly, capitalize on your good experiences as this will not only make your partner feel good but it will also ensure they do the same for you the next time both of you have sex. Try not to sound selfish as you talk about your experience and future expectations. You can do this by using 'we' more than 'I'. Your partner will listen keenly if you make it about both of you rather than yourself.

Tell them how they performed- After telling them how your experience was, now tell them how they performed as well. As much as you need to give an honest opinion, this is one part where you need to tread carefully. Not everybody takes sexual criticism positively, even those that do, they take it with a pinch of salt. Start by lauding their prowess in certain aspects, make them feel like the beast in the bedroom everyone would admire. When you are done complementing them, now gently tell them their weaknesses. How you say it determines the impact those words will have on them. Instead of saying, 'I don't like the way you reached climax fast', you can say. 'It would make me very happy if you could last a little longer next time'. The second statement is still negative but with a better approach than the first. Your partner will likely take it positively and do better in the next round of sex.

Let your partner talk about their experience- make this a two-sided affair by showing an interest in their part of the story. You should also be careful here because your partner might say some things to merely please you. Try not to ask things in a coercive manner. Float to them mind-provoking ideas and questions that would make them start talking automatically. Say things like, 'I saw the way you groaned with pleasure when I touched your butt'. This simple but naughty statement will provoke a response and you will be able to tell whether the groaning was a result of pleasure, discomfort or pain. Always give a response to every statement from your partner. Assure them that you will do the things they like even better next time or you will work on the ones they don't like to enable them to experience better sex in the future.

Talk about the frequency of sex- after both of you have talked about your individual experiences, you now sit down and talk about future sexual encounters. Keep in mind that people are different and the bodies are diverse. Some people will need sex more frequently than others. Talk about the amount of sex the two of you have just had and how long it will take before you need another one. Sex should not be a scheduled thing, yes, but again the frequency of sex matters a lot. You will find that the man will need sex more often than the woman. If you don't work out an interval that works for both of you, one partner might end up straining for the other. We know too well that this kind of scenario will strain the relationship sooner or later.

As a parting shot, communication during the three stages of sex must remain the same. Aim to maintain the status quo before, during and after sex. Communication becomes quite complicated in the last two stages as there is no that intense desire for each other as it was before and immediately when you started having sex. However, the last stage is when both partners get completely honest with each other. No nice things are being said just because you need sex. The point is you should be honest with one another from the beginning to avoid going back on things the two of you agreed on.

Chapter 2: Methods to Trigger Sexual Desire in Your Partner

Sexual desire is an expression of interest in sexual activities and objects. For two people to end up having actual sex, both of them must have a mutual attraction for each other. This must not be confused with love because many people normally end up having sex because they interpret other things such as lust and infatuation as love. However, sexual desire and love can both lead to sex independently but with extremely different results. In the absence of love, sexual desire ends immediately after penetration or other sexual acts and it will take sexual starvation to restore the desire once more. In the case of love, sex is just a fraction of a bigger thing (love) between the participants. However, this desire must always be nourished between couples as it is central to their intimacy. Sex is extremely boring and draining if there is no desire. Desire should come naturally but man has been creative enough to devise ways to provoke it. This requires art and tact to do it successfully. These are the things we are going to highlight in this chapter.

Break of the Routine

To have an overly spicy sex life, always be ready to welcome new stimulations and 'risks' in your bedroom. Sex becomes boring if it is always predictable and uneventful. Most people are afraid of change and that is why they stick to age-old sexual techniques, they feel safer that way. However, the lack of creativity and familiarity breeds contempt. Most cheating couples are the people that no longer find sex interesting in the comfort of their bedrooms. Human beings are naturally programmed to be curious and adventurers. They are always looking for new experiences to feed their curiosity and break the monotony. As partners, make these new experiences readily available in your bedroom by inventing and improvising methods that trigger your sexual appetite for each other. You can do this using the methods below.

Be kids in the bedroom- sexual desire is driven by playfulness around each other. Jump over your partner's shoulders and stick a small note with the words 'I want you' onto their breast pocket. Chase each other around the bedroom completely naked, tease your partner with your nakedness and let them crave for it. Delay actual sexual contact for as long as you can until you are completely sure that they are getting overwhelmed. Creating suspense works wonders when it comes to triggering sexual desire and arousal. Sex starts in the mind, this means that the more fantasies you create the more the desire and the more entertaining it will be when it comes to having sex.

Avoid predictability- offer your partner sex when they least expect. If you are used to having sex after meals, for example, try having it immediately one or both of you come home from work. You can follow them to the shower and strip before they do. First, they will be hit by a surprise before their body quickly embraces it. This makes the sexual experience at that particular unplanned time many times better than during the usual time. Ambush your partner with a variety of toys if they are into them. Bring something that will leave their stay wide open for a couple of minutes, like an oversized dildo, for example. Surprise your partner with the new style in town. Don't be shy to demonstrate it like a pro. This will send their sexual desire through the roof, the same as yours.

Try new things- for once, you can have sex on top of your kitchen table or the couch. Even having it in the woods where no one can see you is equally as thrilling. I am sure that kind of sex will be more thrilling than the one you are used to having in your bedroom. The new environment gives you unmatched pleasure since you will be forced to even improvise the sex position. Just imagine the view and the touch as your bodies get pushed to the limit to stay comfortable. The new adventure might take unusually long and this means more pleasure for the two of you. You can find ideas for new locations and positions of lovemaking from a variety of sources including X-rated movies and books. Make sure every sexual encounter is unique and different from the previous one, even by the slightest thing as slapping your partner's butt. Notice how they react to the new things and know which ones to keep and which ones to discard.

Choose a Sensually appealing environment- take all your five senses into account when selecting the location to have sex. Also, make sure the place appeals to your partner for maximum pleasure. Look for the sweetest-smelling perfume and apply it to every corner of your bedroom. Spread your bed with sheets that send sexual goosebumps all over your body. You can go the extra mile by spreading some beautiful petals on it. This serves as a message to whoever sets their foot in that place, your partner. Make sure the walls are painted in the most romantic colour as well. If you think your bedroom is not an ideal place for this purpose, you can improvise and look for someone else, say a hotel room in a serene environment or a room overlooking the balcony where there is plenty of fresh air. When it comes to the sense of touch, you can use a scarf with soft fur to caress your partner until they get aroused. Also, caress yourself seductively as this also works for you and your partner. If the two of you like listening to music, play soft romantic songs just before and during sex. This helps to elevate your moods and desire for each other. Also, run your tongue through objects in the presence of your partner. This sends sexual signals to them and helps in their arousal. This must not be too hard as well, a simple thing like licking your lips or the edge of your cup works wonders.

Reduction of Sources of Stress

One of the biggest roles of sex is to free you from stress and anxiety. However, stress can crawl on you during sex and spoil the fun. Always aim at avoiding all these kind of distractions during sex as they will not only interfere with the activity during that particular time but also destroys future encounters. The following tips will help you handle stress during sex.

Speak your mind- most stresses accumulate as a result of an individual is unwilling to talk about their issues. People are afraid of revealing their problems because they don't want to be judged. However, things are quite different when it comes to couples. There is no better person to open your heart to than the person you love. They should be the ones that know all your secrets and solve your problems when they can. The good thing about handling stress is that it can reduce when an individual just talks about it. Open your heart and pour out all your problems immediately you arrive home. Your partner will listen and that alone will make you feel better. When it comes to sex, your mind will be clear and you will be able to concentrate.

Show love and compassion to your partner- another effective way of dealing with stress is by having alternative thoughts rather than the stressful ones. If you love your partner, then you should know that they come first no matter the situation. Stress should be the last thing that comes between you and your partner. A simple act of kissing will is enough to prevent your mind from wandering. Tell yourself that it is time for you and your partner and not a time to entertain destructive thoughts. Repeat this statement to yourself every time you feel stressed until your concentration is fully restored.

Stay connected in all aspects- when having sex, ensure your presence is felt by your partner physically, emotionally and mentally. Again, this ensures that your mind is not left idle to wander off. Connect with your partner in a way that makes you feel relaxed and peaceful. Find comfort in the beauty of their presence.

Find a common ground- some stress might come up when you are with your partner. This kind of stress arises from disagreements or arguments. In such a scenario, always take your partner's side and not the opposition. Competing will only spoil the fun you two are having or are about to have. Issues can always be ironed out after sex, just not in the course of it. Respect the moment and get the most out of it.

Learn to listen- if you two are having a light argument, let each one of you talk about their concerns before the other one takes over. Ensure the argument does not escalate because one partner is not listening to the other. You'd rather let the argument become a stalemate than throwing away the fun that's right before you. Be assured that you do not enjoy the sex with the bitterness of having lost an argument.

Get enough rest- sex is a demanding and vigorous activity that uses up most of your energy including that of the mind. Stress only serves to makes things worse if you engage in sexual activity when you are tired. Ensure you have some good rest a few minutes or hours before sex. If you are from work, for example, spend the first few minutes to rest. You can also grab some sleep to help your mind relax. This ensures that you don't end up having sex with a lot of baggage. If you make the mistake of not getting enough rest before sex, you will be looking forward to the end of it rather than enjoying the moment.

Eat well- a healthy balanced diet is another powerful stress reliever that you need to look into. Take your sexuality into consideration before putting food on that plate. Some foods are known to boost your libido and energy. Include a lot of fruits and vegetables in your everyday diet as these two are good at reducing stress. Instead of eating one huge meal at a go, break it into several small meals taken at several intervals. This ensures a consistent supply of energy to your body.

Always put on a smile- a smile doesn't have to be genuine for it to work. Just smile long enough and your brain will pick up the signal. It will interpret the fake smile as genuine and release hormones of happiness. These hormones will radiate to other parts of the body and suppress stress in the process. You can also induce happiness by watching a comedy show or by reading an interesting book, whatever it takes for you to plant that smile on your face.

Don't pay too much attention to orgasms
Reaching an orgasm puts way too much unnecessary pressure

on a couple, especially a woman. If you want to have fulfilling sex, take orgasms off the table completely. An orgasm happens because you have had maximum pleasure and not because you have worked for it. Some orgasms come in less than five minutes while others come after almost thirty minutes. Still, some people do not experience them at all. If you keep your mind fixed to only attaining an orgasm, you will end up forgetting even more important things such as the calm and relaxation that comes with sex. Long and fulfilling sex is equally good as an orgasm. Also, there is some sort of disappointment that comes with not getting what you hoped for. In this case, an orgasm. This is additional stress that is uncalled for. Just enjoy the sex and the orgasm will automatically come, it cannot be forced.

Clear all sexual blocks

Sex with a previous partner might have given you a different perspective about sex. These past experiences must not interfere with your sex life whatsoever. Understandably, some sexual traumas such as rape or injury are hard to forget but you have to give it a shot. Convince yourself that this time around is different, you are doing it with someone you love and it will remain that way. Some obstacles are culture-based, those should be done away with too. Some communities have taught people that sex is meant for procreation alone, don't let that hinder you. Human beings and dolphins are the only organisms that have sex for fun in addition to procreation, keep that in mind too. Don't hide behind the curtain when it comes to sex. Having a high libido, for example, is normal and no one will crucify you for that. If at all you think that is a problem, confirm with a sex therapist and they will tell you the same thing, as long as that doesn't interfere with other areas of your life. People that openly display their sexuality, not to the public, are overly attractive and appealing. It is a way of improving your desire for sex with your partner.

Resumption of physical activity

Aspire to connect with your physical body as a way of triggering your sexual desire. Keep in mind that sex is preceded by physical activity and must be treated as such. Bodily exercise is the most effective way to reconnect with your body. A physically fit body is the most sexually appealing object you will ever find. Fitness reduces stress and enhances your desire for sex. Also, physical activity provides the body with energy to have mind-blowing sex. I will not emphasize the fact that a physically active body is quite flexible when it comes to sex. Having a fit body does not necessarily mean going to the gym. You can decide to go for a walk in the evenings. Another effective way of reconnecting with yourself physically is to Pilates while doing a less strenuous exercise like cooking or watching a movie.

Visit a massage parlour and have your muscles worked once in a while. You can also massage yourself at home, slowly and gently until you feel better. Masturbate regularly, not necessarily to achieve an orgasm but just to burn up that extra fat. Masturbation gives you more experience with your body in terms of fitness and sexually, just don't overdo it.

Having a cold or warm shower is also a way of reconnecting with your body physically. Apart from the physical relief, you will also be released from stress and anxiety. Every time the water hits your bare skin, a whole load of stress leaves your head. When you come out of that shower, you will feel a new wave of energy and sexual desire sweep through you.

Do these bodily exercises daily and it will become a habit before you know it, and your desire for sex will increase each time you reconnect with yourself through physical activity.

Chapter 3: Erotic Massage: When to Use It and Bases on How to Practice It

Erotic massage is a unique type of massage that focuses on the partner's erogenous zones. When done appropriately, erotic massage leads to increased intimacy and provides stress relief to either of the partners. The term "erotic" means Eros, which is a Greek word for love, describing the arousal of intense desire or sexual feelings. Eroticism can be introduced to almost anything that you do -be it eating a meal, dancing, or listening to music -to get in touch with your earthly sexual nature by engaging all your senses.

Erotic massage uses sexual energy to intensify sexual fulfillment through prolonged pleasure, heightened arousal, and increased intimacy. With erotic massage, the partners feel encouraged to freely express their sexual passion, desire, fantasy, and lust. Erotic massage also comes with healing effects, as the erotic energy flows throughout the body. Both partners end up enjoying the bliss sensation of the erotic touch hence receiving feelings of deep relaxation.

Importance of erotic massage

Clearing your mind

Sometimes life can get hectic as we are always in motion to achieve one thing or another in our daily schedules. Our minds get clogged with a flow of many thoughts. Although there are several other methods such as spa retreats, meditation, and yoga, which can be used to restore mental calm, nothing can be productive like a massage. As your partner's hands move upon your physical form, your attention gets centered on such movements alone, making a massage very a very strong relaxation tool. You only concentrate on enjoying the massage without having to do anything, making your mind to settle and relax for a while.

When you get in such deep relaxation mood, your thought and emotional concerns fall into perspective, making you remember what matters in your life. What makes an erotic massage very powerful its ability to reach for your sexual energy and harness it to your advantage. As your mind gets filled with such erotic energy, it gets cleared of any clutter of clogged thoughts; hence, you end up with feelings of orgasmic pleasure and harmony.

Improving your health

Erotic massage stimulates blood circulation in a very effective manner. You end up feeling supple and physically light, in addition to the deep mental relaxation. This physical lightness comes as a result of reaping the benefits of the blood being transported to your bones, muscles, and all the other body organs in an efficient manner. Through massage, blood is directed to flow quickly into the heart where it gets recharged and pumped again to circulate into the body organs. Massage techniques using strokes such as cupping, hacking, and drumming on your partner's skin stirs up the release of toxic waste that has collected below their skin's surface.

Boosting your relationship

As you massage each other, you are also spending time together in an intimate manner. This helps to foster love, trust, and intimacy. You get time to give each other attention and get the opportunity to explore and appreciate your partner's body, as well as discovering which parts of your partner's body respond more intimately to touch and where he/she holds tension.

Basic massage techniques and how to practice them

- **Flowing:** in this technique, you keep your hands flat, and then sweep them, back and forth over the corners and curves of your partner's body in a long, smooth flowing motion. To keep the pressure evenly spread across your hands and make sure that they slide smoothly without catching, keep the hands well oiled. These long flowing strokes should be used over larger areas of your partner's body such as buttocks, chest, the back, the belly, and the legs.

- **Circling:** in this technique, you keep your hand flat, and then make circles, moving them away from each other, then back again in a circular motion on your partner's skin. This stroke is used on buttocks, belly, back, legs, and chest where there is enough skin for your hands to make opposing circles in a complete way.

- **Mini circles:** this varies slightly from circling. It entails making just small circles using your fingertips. If the area is fleshy, you can press harder with your fingers, than when using the entire hand. This applies best on areas such as the breasts, side of the neck, chest areas, facial cheek muscles and other muscles which carry tension and knots such as upper back and shoulder muscles.

- **Friction:** to stimulate the skin's surface, this technique uses firm and fast rubbing action with both hands. Such rubbing generates heat, which penetrates deeper body areas. Less sensitive areas such as shoulders, legs, buttocks, legs, back, and the arms are best suited for this vigorous stroke.

- **Kneading:** with this technique, you grab a handful of flesh and knead it as if you are kneading the dough for making bread, using your hands and fingers at a relatively rapid pace and with confidence. This stroke works well on any fleshy body areas such as the top of shoulders, calf muscles, waist, upper arms, thighs, belly, and buttocks.

- **Electric socket:** this wobbles the surface of the skin by moving two figures rapidly to create a fast vibrating movement. Areas such as the middle of the lower belly, between the nipples and the forehead, are some of the regions where this stroke works well. It sends a charged feeling thought-out the body of your partner.

- **Thumbing:** keep your hands as flat as possible against your partner's body, and make rapid, small alternate strokes using your thumbs either pushing away or in circles. This stroke is effective when massaging fleshy and muscly areas close to a bone such as the back of the legs, fronts of the thighs, arms, thumbing up either side of the spine and back of the neck.

- **Clawing:** you pull your fingertips towards yourself using fairly firm pressure, one hand after the other. This stroke can be tried on the back, chest, and thighs. Get feedback from your partner on whether you are scratching too hard, especially if you have long nails.

- **Feathering:** create a light featherweight touch using your fingertips by drawing one hand after the other towards you. You can also use an actual sizable, and real feather almost everywhere to trace light touches on your partner's body. You can try it on buttocks, back, legs and shoulders.

- **Flacking:** you rhythmically hack areas with enough flesh using the sides of your hands, to stimulate and excite the body, hence bringing blood to the skin's surface. This stroke works well on buttocks, shoulders, backs of thighs, and at the back, away from the spine.

- **Cupping:** with your hands lightly rounded, alternate them in a drumming action over your partner's skin. This stroke fits well as you move your hands on fleshy body areas such as calf muscles, buttocks, and thighs.

- **Knuckling:** grind into the muscles using your knuckles with your hand in a fist shape. When your partner is lying face down, use this stroke on the lower neck, palms of the hands, the arches of the feet, the back of the legs and buttocks.

- **Draining:** this deep stroke technique works well for the legs and the arms. While holding the arm at the wrist, use both thumbs to press on the inside of the arm. Your thumbs should then slide up towards the elbow, before pulling your flat hands down the sides and the inside of the arm to the hand. For the calf muscles, start at the ankle and do the same as you have done to the arms.

- **Twisting:** this is ideal for the legs and the arms where you use both hands to wring them the same way you wring out a cloth. Using a large, circular, turning action, from the underside to the outside, you can twist your partner's foot with one hand.

- **Licking and biting:** these are unique stokes given using the mouth. You can create lots of pleasurable sensations and erotic charge using your tongue, teeth, or lips. You lick delicate areas with the whole flat or the tip of your tongue, bite fleshy areas gently and nibble with your teeth. You then use your lips to calm the areas with erotic kisses.

Whole-body massage

The purpose of these techniques if to alleviate tensions, boost blood circulation, relax the whole body, and simulate the genitals gently. Rather than trying to force your own speed and rhythm, you work with the natural motion of your partner's body while massaging sensitively, smoothly and confidently. Before you start an erotic body massage, as well as during one, you can try both wiggling and rocking.

Rocking

The aim is to rock your partner like a baby, in a very soothing manner to loosen the tension that holds the body rigid in the joints and the muscles. As the genitals are being pressed against the surface of the mattress, they get stimulated in a gentle way. You take your partner to an erotic sexual peak by arousing them in an unhurried, relaxed style, guiding without pushing.

- Hip rocking: push your partner's body away from you by pushing the hip that is closest to you with your hand, then as the hips roll back to your arms, catch them. Place your hands on her thighs and roll them from side to side to generate a reasonably vigorous motion. After some minutes, change to the other thigh.

- Sacrum rocking: rock your partner's hips from side to side by placing your both hands on her sacrum. Your partner's body will assume a certain natural rhythm which you are supposed to follow. Don't try to force your own rhythm, but try to increase the force of the rocking gradually until it becomes somehow vigorous by following the rhythm of her body.

Wiggling

Both hands are used to shake different parts of the body of

your partner in this dynamic technique. It aims at relaxing the joints, in order to release any tension. It is used with your partner laying on her back.

- **Foot wiggle:** hold your partner's foot with your both hands while she lies on her back. Wiggle the leg by passing it forward and backwards at a fast pace between your two hands. Repeat the same for the other foot to relax tension in the joints of both feet.

- **Shoulder wiggle:** your partner should lie on her back as you sit above her head. Start to push each shoulder towards your partner's feet, wiggling from one hand to another in close succession as you are bouncing a ball on your hands. Of its own accord, your partners head will start to rock from side to side, hence relieving the neck of any tension.

- **Arm wiggle:** you hold your partner's hand and raise it slightly as if you are shaking it. To loosen the arm and shoulder joints, shake the arm from side to side in a vigorous way.

While massaging your partner, slowly incorporate the erogenous zones into the above primary massage techniques. Take the time to explore your partner's body gently and slowly to discover their erogenous zones. Regularly, check-in with your partner at every stage of the massage to ensure that they are comfortable.

Pay attention to both the verbal and non-verbal cues so that you can know what feels excellent for the other partner. You should be free to involve the usage of lubrication and massage oils such as silicone-based oils or water-based lubrication to avoid any form of infection. Sex toys are also fantastic to use throughout the process of erotic massage. Communicate with each other regularly to establish what works best for each one of you.

The aim of all this is to discover the erogenous zones of either partner on the other parts of the body other than their genitals. Always remember that the erotic massage is aimed at providing an alternative source of relaxation pleasure without necessarily having to involve sex or the genitals. Orgasms and ejaculations may come as an essential part of a long process, but they are not necessarily the main focus. After you are done with a full-body massage, you can slowly begin to move to the genitals, to give your partner more sensual pleasure.

Chapter 4: Preliminaries: Their Importance, How To Do Them The Best. What She Prefers and What He Prefers.

There are several things which you can engage in as a couple in preparation for erotic massage. These act as a way of preparing yourselves and setting the environment before you sink yourselves into the arousing each other. When you have a guest, you show them a table which has been prepared to in a unique way for them. This should also apply when you want to give your partner a unique gift of massage. The environment should be prepared beforehand in an attractive manner. A fragrant environment is crucial to create relaxation and comfort by setting the right mood so that your partner gains the optimum benefit from such an exceptional experience.

Setting the environment

You need a sanctuary that will enable you to focus on your time together and forget worries of the outside world so that you can have a genuinely satisfying erotic massage. You may set aside space in your house by choosing either your living space, bedroom, and bathroom, or any other place in the house where you will feel more comfortable. Such a room should be made clean, warm, and welcoming to your partner. By clearing all the clutter in the room, your bodies will start to unwind, and the mind will be able to empty more quickly. You will both have a greater connection and fully gain from the massage when you settle into a peaceful state.

You may use a table to massage some parts of your partner's body, such as legs, back, chest, or shoulders. But you also need a place prepared on the floor or a bed for intimate activities that may follow after that. A mattress on the floor or a firm bed will be excellent for this.

Use freshly laundered sheets and towels

Have cleaned sheets or towels which a freshly washed to cover your partners with or for them to lie on. Everything that you use, ranging from throws, blankets, sheets, towels, or cushions, should be smell freshly laundered and clean.

Lighting

To evoke an atmosphere for sensuality, calm and relaxation, use candlelight and muted light. Place the candles in safe areas where they cannot be knocked down in such a way that they pool the place of the massage in soft light. Change your routinely used bulbs and experiment with coloured ones to create an instant change to the atmosphere of that room. To bath your bodies with warm, flattering light, soften the hard edges, and suffuse the room with a pink hue, a red bulb will your best choice.

Temperature

The room should be warm and draft-free to prevent your partner from feeling cold when the massage oils begin to evaporate from the surface of the skin. Drafts become more noticeable when you lie close to the ground, especially when you decide to massage close to a door. Coldness on the skin can make it hard to relax as it may begin to contract fully. You may incorporate the use of a fan to bring a cooling effect if the room is somehow hot. This will help to keep your partner awake and counteract any hypnotic effect of the massage.

Aroma

In a state of relaxed awareness, can bring a powerful effect on someone as it is highly evocative. It can bring a profound relaxation effect by uniquely transporting the mind. Throughout the massage period, you can burn essential oils using an oil diffuser, by choosing oils that match or complement the ones you are applying for the massage. If you wish to burn incense but ensure that it is made of natural ingredients as synthetic incense can overwhelm you in your small space. To avoid harmful chemicals, you can also bring soft light and fragrance in the room by using scented candles.

Oils and lubricants

You need to choose natural oils that will not irritate your partner's skin such as light olive oils, grape-seed, or almond. To add aroma, you need to use a few drops of these essential oils. Some of the scents excellent for erotic massage are:

- Lavender, which helps in relaxation

- Jasmine absolute – relieves sexual tension and enlivens male sexuality.

- Rose absolute –this promotes a feeling of love

- Neroli absolute –soothes anxiety and stimulates fertility/virility

- Sandalwood, which increases feelings of calm and sensuality

Use a bowl of recently boiled water to warm the oils before you begin. As you continue the massage, regularly replenish your hands with the oil, and keep the oil warm by returning the oil bottle to the bowl. Use water-based lubricants made purposely for intimate use for intimate genital massage. Ovoid using oils internally as they can cause infection or irritation.

Toys and tools

You will find several toys that you can buy in the market to enhance your erotic massage experience. Here are a few examples:

- Water spray bottle – it has a battery to power its functionality

- Vibrator – this is excellent for use on the whole body.

- Feather duster, feathers or feather fan

- Silk shawl or sarong with tassels

Privacy

Privacy is vital. You want to make sure that you will not have and interruption or disturbance throughout the massage session. Switch off your phones, and if you have little children, make sure that they are asleep or are out of the reach of your room. If your children are older or teenagers, tell them that you are in for a massage session and they will stay away. Put a notice on the front door so that visitors will be aware that you are resting and they should not ring the bell.

Music

Music is a great way to mask any unwelcome sounds coming from outside, as well as evoking an erotic mood. You can play ambient music that is written explicitly for massage, which is not too insistent or invasive. Choose a long playlist so that you won't need to rise to change it.

Environment

Make an effort to acquire exquisite towels, sheets, rugs, cushions, and shawls to create an environment where your partner will fee pampered to enrich the massage session experience as much as possible. Enhance the mystery and the magic of the massage by surrounding your space with romantic materials in luxurious colours.

You can also schedule your massage session outside if the weather is warm and you have a secluded yard outside. Take advantage of the proximity of nature to enrich your massage experience. Things like the singing of the birds, the sound of the wind brazing via the trees .water running into a bowl and the sun caressing your skin can revolutionize the massage experience. Carry water to drink if the sun is hot and some shawl or blanket to cover your partner in case the sun gets too hot or the weather becomes chilly.

Establish ground rules

- Discuss with your partner before trying new things so that you can establish boundaries and understand each other's expectation. This will enable you to know the likes of your partner and the dos and dons during the massage session as you seek to try new things. Understanding each other's perspective will make it possible for you to approach the session with confidence.

- Pay attention to what is happening to your partner's body as a way to show honour and respect to them. You will be able to notice the touches which they enjoy the most and spend more time there before moving on to another area. Don't allow anything to distract you during the massage session. If your partner shows any signs of discomfort or reacts negatively to particular touches during the massage session, agree to respond immediately and make adjustments.

- Remember this is not about what you think is good, but what your partner likes and enjoys the most. So, you must respond positively even if you cannot understand why your partner is not enjoying touches which you think are great. If your partner is not comfortable being touched on some areas of the body, be careful to avoid them.

- Don't talk unnecessarily. Allow the session to be calm so that your partner can relax. Unless it has been agreed beforehand, don't try to manoeuvre your partner to such things as penetrative sex, towards orgasm or any other goal.

Prepare yourself for the massage.

Mental and physical preparation is essential. Take a shower before the massage session, relax your mind, control your breathing and cleanse, and pamper your bodies.

Expressing your love

- Hugs and embraces –before and after the massage session, embrace your partner with a heart-to-heart full-bodied hug to reinforce mutual trust between the two of you.

- Caresses: communicate your desires, fascination, and appreciation to your partner thought caresses. You can do this before the massage, during the massage or after the massage.

- Kisses: make time to kiss each other beforehand to promote emotional connection, romance, and intimacy. Pause to kiss your partner during the massage on the lips and other sensitive parts of the body.

- Bathing your partner: to promote feelings of emotional and physical intimacy, showering is an excellent way. You can shower your partner before and after the massage session in a relaxed and yet erotic way.

- Play erotic games: before the massage session, take some time and engage in playing erotic and creative games together. Your mind will let go of any and allow your body to be more responsive, more spontaneous, and more accessible to touch. The sense of laughter and fun which comes with such games will also play a key role in helping to put aside your cares.

- Get outside for a change: break the boredom by changing your typical environment. This helps to create impromptu and spontaneous, playful moments. Visit a secluded garden, a place in the woods, or an unfrequented beach to get in touch with nature. Eat delicious foods that you do not take routinely. Feed each other in an erotic sensual manner as you get in touch with such a natural moment with all your senses.

Sensual woman

Women are aroused differently from men, and it may take time to understand what your partner wants to be simulated. You should take your time to understand and appreciate your partner's responses so that you can understand their needs and desires.

Female erogenous areas

There are some specific zones which you should focus on to make your partner respond more intimately to your touch. There are some erogenous zones which are common for both men and women. To arouse and delight your female partner, focus on the following parts.

- Lips –lips will respond more intimately to gentle strokes using your fingertips and kissing in different ways.

- Neck –the sides of the neck produce very erotic feelings for your partner when stroked and nibbled.

- Hands –for an erotic charge, suck the fingertips and stroke palms of gently with your fingertips.

- Arms –for delicious sensation, stroke the inside of the lower arm gently using the tips of your fingers.

- Breasts –touch and caress the whole breast area, which is highly sensitive. Give more attention to the nipples when she is aroused.

- Waist –you can knead this sensitive, erogenous area using both hands or use your fingertips to stroke it.

- Lower belly – to arouse her sexual appetite, massage this erogenous area, including the pubic hairline.

Caressing her erogenous zones

Erotic massage is a great way to help you discover your partner's erogenous zones as you caress the different part of the body. When you touch an erogenous zone, she becomes more sensitive and accompanies such sensitivity with new erogenous responses. As you caress her, you will enjoy getting closer to her sensual curves and the responses she will have as you move your hands on her body.

- Both of you should close your eyes as your partner lies comfortably. Tune into her breathing so that both of you breathe in and out together as you rest your hands on her belly.

- Caress her curves using one hand. As you stroke her, you may get aroused as you do so, but restrain yourself from lead her to having sex so that she can fully enjoy the massage. Listen to any sounds that point to her arousal and pleasure by keeping your breathing low.

- For a moment, stop the movement of your hand when you sense that you are caressing or stroking an erogenous zone, and use your fingers to trace the lines over that area.

- Using your mouth, kiss, and lick the erogenous zone slowly and gently as you breathe warm air in the region. As you do this, continue exploring her with both of your hands to find another erogenous zone to excite and caress.

Sensual man

To draw out and develop a man's sensual nature, erotic massage is an excellent and effective way. Erotic massage can help to eliminate any form of resistance a man may have and reveal his sensual and softer side. When this happens, you should encourage him to relax and enjoy it as you continue to caress him with love and awareness.

Accessing a man's sensual nature

When it comes to sensuality, men are different creatures from women and tend to be less intuitive and more practical. They use the analytical right side to process the happenings of the real world other than the emotional left side. For a man to explore his sensuality fully, he must willingly let go of his sense of order so that he can get in touch with his sensual side. To help a man release his potent sensual energy, erotic massage is a powerful tool.

To access a man's sensual nature easily, go through his mind because men are visual creatures. They have a particular appetite for simulating materials that are pleasing to the eye, such as proactive lingerie and erotic dancing. Men are also sensitive to audio input. When a man hears the voice of a lover or listens to auditory erotic literature, he can connect with his sensual side. To make your male partner get absorbed totally to the sensuality of the moment, you should learn to incorporate these elements into your erotic massage.

The ultimate pleasure zone

The centre of a man's sexuality is his genitals. By exploring this ultimate erogenous zone of a man, you can both have a lot of fun. Such erotic areas include the perineum, penis, and scrotum. The perineum is the area between the anus and the scrotum. Being an ending of highly sensitive nerve, the genital region of the male is the hotbed of is eroticism.

Therefore erogenous zones can produce remarkable sensation and pleasure when touched and massaged in the right manner. These sensitive body regions can be explored through touch as you press your partner's body slowly and gently. As you massage your partner, you should avoid pursuing your selfish interest such as trying to manoeuvre them to orgasm or towards penetrative sex, unless you had planned it before. Remember that erotic massage doesn't have to involve orgasm and ejaculations, although they can be a happy ending if they come as a result of a long process.

Chapter 5: Ten Pleasant Positions for Both

Sex can have an array of aims depending on the partners. The aims for having sex include pleasure, a celebration of a milestone in your relationship, having a child or even to mark a resolution to a previous disagreement. Apart from that, sex can also be used as a way of bringing couples together and make them value each other and strengthen their bond. Sex can be viewed as different things depending on an individual. It can be slightly awkward, pleasant, adventurous, full of giggles and erotic among many other views. Sex can be done slowly in a luxurious manner or super speedy usually depending on the situation and the couple's preferences.

Sex is an act that can be executed in various postures, positions, and styles. Some of these sex positions and styles are so complicated while others are easy. Some are pleasant to both partners while others are only pleasant to one and sour to another. Some of these positions are done with partners facing each other while others not. There is an array of sex styles with different executive positions. In this article, we are going to focus on a few sex positions that are pleasant to both partners and not complicated either. These sex positions are the most intimate and we have preferred face to face positions. They include;

- **Spooning**

Spooning is one of the easiest sex positions that anyone can do. There are various spooning positions which are executed in different ways. They include the serving spoon, the silver spoon, spoon dog, slotted spoon and the spoon river. We are not going to look into these spooning positions but rather the inverted spoon position. An inverted spoon position is a form of spooning sex posture whereby the woman faces the male partner rather than facing away as in other spooning positions. In this position, the man lies on his side with the woman also lying facing him. The woman then slightly spreads her legs to allow the man to penetrate her. She then closes in her legs such that some part of the man's penis is outside her vagina and can caress the clitoris. At this position, thrusting may not be very easy and thus the couple should use different approaches such as circular motion and grind. In this position, linear thrusting is not advisable and the up-and-down thrusting is the most appropriate.

This sex position is very pleasant to both partners as one partner does not have to bear the other's weight at any time. It also favours instances where one partner has an injury that does not allow them to bear the body's weight. This position is also so intimate as the couple will get time to face each other and read each other's feelings. Since the partners are facing each other, it will be easy for them to be kissing each other at the same time they are penetrating each other. This will be an added advantage for even more pleasure.

- **Side to Side**

The side to side sex position is another variation of the spooning sex position. This sex position is a favour to individuals who have huge bodies and finds the spooning position complicated for them. In this position, both partners lay side by side facing each other. Depending on the sex type one is having, the positions and approaches taken vary. If you are having anal sex, the woman will have to just lean forward and backwards while either straightening or bending their legs. In this position, the woman can be able to rub themselves to get an orgasm as the man penetrates her when having anal sex.

In the side to side position, the man can easily penetrate the woman slowly and luxuriously. This position is also pleasing to both partners since the woman can be able to caress herself or the man with ease during sex. On the other hand, both partners can even find time to easily kiss while having sex thus get whole pleasure. While penetrating, the man can choose to go slow or fast to allow the partners to have longer intimate experience thus an increased pleasure to both partners. In this position, the partners will also get a good time to strongly bond and strengthen their relationship thus making it so intimate and pleasurable.

- **Woman on top**

This is a sex position where the man lay on his back then the woman takes control on the top. This sex position is more playful as compared to any other and accrues some distinct advantages. At this position, the woman gets symbolic and visceral control than when she is underneath. The woman can control the depth and speed of the penetration making it more to her liking. This proves to be very simple and without any complications, since the woman can be able to do it all without having to order the man to either go faster, slower or harder. In this way, the woman will most likely get orgasm easily and in a more pleasurable manner. At this position, the man has nothing much to do but just enjoy the pleasure.

This position is like a form of reversed coital alignment technique. Women enjoy this position since they get a variety of positions while on top of the man. The woman in this position should position herself in such a way that her clitoris gets into contact with the pubic bone of her man. This will ensure that she gets high clitoral stimulation which will trigger an orgasm and great pleasure. At this point, the man has nothing much to do. He can only grind against you gently thus making the whole thing more interesting and fascinating. Apart from that, the man can support the woman's hips with his hands thus helping her thrust upwards and downwards. This position is the easiest with no complications. The fact that both partners maintain a face to face contact makes it a very intimate and pleasurable position.

- **Mixed missionary**

A mixed missionary sex position is disliked by many due to its tendency of being basic and boring but the truth is that this position is classic in some way. Although it is disliked by some people, this position remains one of the simplest and easiest. One of the partners lies and does nothing while the other person on top does all the work. In many cases, the lady is the one who lies down while the man stays on the top doing all that concerns the sex process. It is also suitable for newbies because of its simplicity. The person on top, usually the man, controls the depth and power of thrusting as the one below can be moving about their legs and hips to bring about different sensations.

Mixed missionary position has different and numerous variations. This position can be mixed up by simply positioning your legs in different ways. Some modifications can be done such as the partner below placing their legs over the arms of the other person on top. This will help in opening up the woman's vulvo-vaginal area. This will make penetration pleasurable and will allow both partners to get different sensations of pleasure. This position is one of the most romantic sex positions since it entails eye gazing, skin-to-skin contact and smooching. This makes it so intimate and at the same time pleasurable to both partners.

- **Crab**

A crab sex position is another easy sex position which is somehow the same as the woman on top position. In this position, the man lays on her back facing up while the woman stays on top and her knees. The woman will tend to be leaning backwards during penetration such that she bends her man's penis backwards. The woman should ensure that they stretch their hands behind to remain stable in this position. At the same time, the man should ensure that he keeps his legs together. This position also needs the man to make sure that he has good penile flexibility due to the bending so that it does not make it complicated.

In the crab position, the woman should lean backwards and support herself on the bed using her hands. When positioning herself, she should be careful to be slow enough to ensure that she does not over-strain his man's penis. Once in the perfect position, she has to thrust her body up and down slowly with the aid of her legs. The woman can also be able to grind the man by moving her hips backwards and forwards in relatively slow motion. On the other hand, the man should always make sure that he is comfortable and enjoys himself without any much pressure on his penis. He can decide to hold onto your hips and move them back and forth as you grind him. This sex position is so intimate since it entails both partners facing each other. It is also a very easy style to execute as it has no major complications if it is done in the right way.

- **Fusion**

A fusion sex position is similar to the crab position but the only difference is that infusion, the partner underneath sits up and leans on a wall or hardboard. The other partner will be thrusting up and down while facing the partner. This position is very easy to execute and it allows one to reach spots during penetration that makes it even more pleasurable. With such pleasure, this makes this position very erotic. The man is usually the one at the bottom while the woman stays on top. Then man crosses his legs while leaning on his hands. The woman will then sit on the top facing his man and then stretch out her legs and also lean on her hands.

In this position, the women will be the one in control. This, therefore, means that she will be the one to dictate the depth and speed of penetration. Many women like this style because it is easy and allows them to get slow sex. Women usually get aroused slower compared to men who get an orgasm very fast thus slow sex would be important for them. This sex position will thus enable the woman to have the sex she desires and get an orgasm which is a pleasure and fascinating sensation to them. The position is also very intimate since both partners maintain eye contact which makes them understand each other and how they feel. It is, therefore, an easy and pleasing sex position to both partners engaging in sex.

- **Victory**

A victory sex position is where the woman lays on a bed or any flat surface then the man stretches the woman's legs apart such that they form a V-shape. During sex employing this style, it is necessary to have a pillow below the woman's head such that she can see what is happening. To get into this position, the lady lies down then extends her legs up such that they form a v-shape. The man will then kneel in front of the woman and position himself at the pelvis of the woman and penetrate her. Once in this position, the man may lean forward using his arms assuming a position as if ready to strike deep. The woman can control the penetration by placing her hands on the man's chest such that she can easily control the depth of penetration.

This position is so intimate since both partners are facing each other during the act. What makes this position laced with great pleasure is that when the woman spreads her legs to form a V-shape, she opens up her vagina to allow deep penetration. This means that the man will be able to thrust without any distractions thus great pleasure. The woman can also control the man such that she gets the sex that she desires thus more pleasure. This position is also very easy to execute and thus can be done by anyone. This position, therefore, qualifies into the list of sex positions that are not complicated and enables both partners to get enough pleasure.

- **Cowboy**

Cowboy sex position has no much difference with the cowgirl sex position. The only difference is that the cowboy is the opposite of the cowgirl position. When having sex using this style, the woman lays underneath while the man is usually on top. The women will lie flat and ensure that their legs are put together. The work of then will, therefore, be straddling the woman and sit on her legs then go down with her penis to enter into the woman. To make it easier for penetration, the woman can slightly raise her hips. The man will also have to adjust his position by moving either backwards or forwards to find the best position in which both of them can get stimulated comfortably without straining anyone of them.

In the cowboy position, the man does almost every work that pertains to the sexual practice. The man is the one to execute the thrusting and ensure that it is as comfortable as possible. When the man gets a perfect positioning in this style, then this will provide maximum stimulation to the woman's clitoris. On the other hand, the woman does very little. She just has to enjoy the penetration and slightly spread her legs to make work easier for his man. The woman may also slightly raise her hips to open up her vagina and allow deeper penetration. This sex position is one of the simplest and allows both partners to get sufficient pleasure without any complications. It is also very intimate and fascinating.

- **Simple scissors**

The scissors sex position is one of the simplest to perform during sex. To perform this position, both partners should first lay side by side such that one leg is on top of the other. The woman will then slightly raise the top leg to allow the man to easily access the vagina. With the man also in the same position, h should ensure that he slips into you thus his head will be close to your feet. He will then place his leg on top of yours and start penetrating you. This means that you will have your underneath leg between your man's legs. You will now lie facing each other but far from each other thus he can just thrust after penetrating you.

In this sex position, the woman should also engage in thrusting by gently moving back and forth as the man is thrusting. On the other hand, the man may grab your leg to help him in thrusting and penetrating deeper. Newbies should use this position as it is easy and carters for the pleasure of both partners. This position ensures that both partners get pleasure since they both engage in thrusting. It is also very simple and has no major complications thus an intimate position.

Chapter 6: Ten Positions Dedicated Mainly To Her, To Give Her Pleasure and Facilitate Orgasm

The aim of sex is for pleasure and also childbearing in most cases. Sex is bound to be good for the two parties that are in it. So how does one achieve pleasure in a woman? This is simply since she has to be comfortable and feel like she is loved. She has to feel like she is at the centre of attention. The woman has to feel like someone is really taking care of her. There are different positions during sex that can make a woman feel pleasure and at the end for her to orgasm.

The first position is what is known as the missionary position. This is the most common position for most people who are sexually active. It is the most basic position and most people start with it. It is comfortable for both parties who are partaking in this activity. This position is very simple and the most natural of all the sex positions. It is simple to carry out and ensures that one gets the end product of pleasure and orgasms. This position is manifested as the man being on top of the woman. The woman gives the manned space between her hips. The space that is provided with the man positions himself on top of her. Here in this position the man is the one who is in charge and should lead the way until the end. This position makes the woman feel like she is sexy and she needs to feel like that for pleasure to kick in. so what happens is that the male makes the woman feel like she is a damsel in distress being saved. This position should not be done from the beginning of the sex till the end. So if you want your woman to feel pleasure and great orgasms then this is the position to take into consideration. It can be done by anyone who wills it.

The next position is what is known as the girl on top. As the name says it the woman is usually on the top. This is usually the opposite of what comes in the missionary position. In this position, the woman is in control of what is going on at the moment. This is usually done by women who like control but also any woman can pull it off. If a woman is allowed to take control during sex she will feel the sense of freedom when it comes to sex. If the woman feels like this sense of freedom then pleasure will kick in so fast. So once in a while, the woman is supposed to take charge of what happens during sex. So how is the girl on top achieved? The first thing to note is that the man should lie below then the woman should come at the top. The man should lie in a prostrate manner. The woman comes to the top near his sexual area where she should set herself in a comfortable manner. This will work if the woman moves her hips during sex. This makes a woman feel like there is a new thing that is around. Here the woman does a lot of work all around. The man can place his hands around the woman's hips. This helps to guide her and also to help her so that she does not get too tired.

Another position is g-whiz. This is a position that is very nice for people who are flexible. This refers to the woman. The people who mostly do this position are either used to doing yoga or even ballerinas. If you are not really flexible this then is not a position you should really take into consideration. So this is the right position to take if you know you can handle a lot of stretching happening on your body. The position that is being discussed allows the man to reach the g-spot which allows the woman to feel pleasure and to finally orgasm. If it is not hit then pleasure is the last thing you are to expect. In this position, the man can easily reach the g-spot of a woman. This position comes to be where the woman can place her legs on top of her head. This is possible when the woman is lying down then the lifting of the legs follow. The man can set the woman's legs on his shoulders to make the woman be totally comfortable during the process. So at the end of it, all this position is great for people who have full-body coordination. The man is in charge when it comes to this position and he is the one who guides the whole process of sex. If you are looking for something to pleasure your woman then this is the right position to do.

The other position suitable to pleasure a woman is the famous doggy style. This is one of the most common types of sex positions in the world. Most women like this style very much and for them, they see it as if it works wonders for their sex life. With this one, the man is able to go deep into the woman. It enables both parties to get to feel so much pleasure. So the point of this position is an easy and deep penetration of the man into the woman. This position comes about as a woman bends down into the position in which looks like the way a dog walks or stands. The man goes behind the woman and there he kneels and sets himself in a manner where he is close to her sexual area. This position and how it comes to be is where the name is from. Most people think it is easy and that it can be done by anyone. The woman can bend her back further for her to be more comfortable as the position makes one feel some sort of abdominal pressure. Women are so receptive to this position and men should know how it is amazing to do it with their sexual partner. If you really want your woman or her to be satisfied and to end up having an orgasm then try this position and see how it goes for you.

The bridge is the position the suits anyone looking to pleasure the woman. It is a very easy position that one can carry out during their sexual activity. It is almost similar to what is the missionary position. It requires the woman to lie down but in this case, she will not just lay flat over there. The man will position himself in front of the woman but in the middle of her hips. Here the man will kneel for this to actually work. This is a little bit different from the missionary position since the man has to give support to the man. Missionary position is the basis of this bridge position for sex. So to know this position you must go back to this basic missionary position in the sex department. The man is supposed to put his hands at the lower back of the woman. This is to offer some kind of place that he can hold on to. With this type of position, the man gets to penetrate deeper and he is able to reach the g-spot with much ease. So in this position, the woman and the man will both get satisfied at the end of it all. So if you are a guy and you are looking to get a woman to feel so much pleasure and orgasm at it then you should do this position.

The L position is the next position too. This is basically said in the name. The letter that is made in this position is the letter L. This position is almost similar to the doggy style. There is a difference between the doggy style and this position here since the woman instead of positioning themselves in a dog walking style the woman lies on the side. After the woman has lied on their side then the man goes behind her and kneels. Here he positions himself near the sexual area of the woman who is his partner. The man then positions the woman's leg into an L letter. In this position, the woman is comfortable without having to kneel and bend their backs. This is very uncomfortable for the woman and this position, therefore, makes the woman's work easy. Remember for pleasure to be found there must be a lot of comfortability. So this position has readily provided that. The L position also allows the man to penetrate more than in most sex position, therefore, it is really a good position. It also allows the man to hit the woman's g-spot just like in the doggy style position. If one needs to make the woman sexually satisfied you can always trust that this position. It makes the pleasure for the woman intense and undeniable and the woman will be able to orgasm even if she has never gone through it before.

The other position is what is known as the scissors position. This is basically as easy as it sounds. Here the man and the woman position themselves in a manner in which both of them make a scissors shape. Here the woman and the man's legs intertwine. One leg of the man goes on top of the woman and so does one leg of the woman. The woman has to lie down as the man is on the other side of her. Here the man can lift himself as he is doing it with the lady. This is actually a good thing since there will be a change during the activity. The other thing that makes this also very good is the fact that the man will be able to penetrate the woman as best as she can. This makes the man reach the g-spot which we have seen having a thing with pleasure and orgasms in a woman. This position is not too comfortable but it has good results coming with it. This sex position makes everything in sex to be more interesting more than other sex positions. The reason why is because most of these positions are the same old basic ones and this one can be the new sizzle in the relationship. So this a great position to take on with your woman. This helps to increase pleasure and get rid of the same old techniques.

The flat iron is the other position. This one is nice for all those who are fans of the doggy style. This is almost the same as the doggy style but is a little comfortable than it. For this position, the woman does not have to suffer around the knee area and also with the back. Here the woman has to sit back and relax and enjoy all that comes with this position. The man is the one in charge in this case and the woman gets to have the fun. The pleasure in this position comes in for both the man and the woman in this case. So how does this position come about to be? This is easy since the woman will just lie with her front side. After that, the mangoes behind her and the woman has to make room in between her hips for the man. The man has to kneel in between her hips and ensure that he has reached a point where he can do the activity very well. This is an easy style that ensures that the woman is not tired. It is the best alternative for the doggy style. If you want the woman comfortable and pleased at the end of the process then one should follow through with this position. For this position whatever is achieved in the doggy style, it is also achieved in this one too.

Another position is what is known as the reverse cowgirl. This position is where one woman is on top of the man. Some people believe that this position is really a good one for both parties to feel pleasure. Here the woman is in charge as she at the top of things. This position is from the riding of cows or even horses. It looks like it has Texas slap to it. So this position, how does it really take place? The first thing is that the man will lay flat and the woman will climb on top of him. The most important thing to know is that the girl or woman will not be facing the man but will be looking in the opposite direction to the place the man's face is. The woman is to set herself on the man's sexual area. Here the woman feels in charge and full of power and authority too. She feels free that she gets to be at the top and has power over the man that is underneath her. So this position is free and liberating. It is also nice if one wants to have a good time, especially in women. It allows the woman to get the man to reach her g-spot which is easy in this case. She becomes the guide and the man is just but an observer in this case. So if you are looking for something to work for you then you can totally take on this position.

Finally, there is the cradle. This is basically the two parties holding each other. The name suggests a lot about what to expect from this position. The man sits then he holds the woman on top of himself. The woman faces him with her legs on both sides for it to work. This is a romantic position and it gives someone the bond that is required for sex to work. This position allows the two parties to get the feel and in the process, both they end up feeling satisfied. This position works for the woman as it allows that she feels so loved and that someone is paying attention to her. Also, the care she is given by the man is fully shown. So at the end in this position both of them are equals. There are so many positions that can be used by you to make a woman get to her orgasm point. These positions above are just but a few. Make a woman not fake an orgasm or having some pleasure at the end of it all. So all the above can be used by you to make sex for the woman something that she can look forward to at the end of the day. So much more has been left out but this is the most basic and easy positions that you can take up for the pleasure and the amusement of the woman.

Chapter 7: Ten Positions Dedicated Mainly To Him, To Give Him Pleasure and Facilitate Orgasm

In this chapter, we take a close look at some of the sex positions that will greatly boost a man's likelihood or ability to have the strongest and most intense climax. In as much as most of these sex positions focus primarily on exploiting the man's sexual organ for maximum pleasure, others are solely meant to boost a man's sexual intimacy with his partner. You might have mastered all these positions but it is vital to make it clear to you that the secret lies in the precision. Paying attention to detail is what changes a normal random bedroom activity to an over the roof pleasure experience. These sex positions will press his buttons in a way that is mind-blowing.

The lusty leapfrog

How to do it effectively

The man should lie on his back facing the ceiling after which the woman should position herself on the tip of the man with her legs on both sides of the man's hips. Thereafter, the woman should gradually lower herself onto his mid-section, sliding his manhood into the vagina as she goes down. However, instead of assuming a sitting position, the woman should raise herself from the man and consequently assume a squatting position. This position might get a little bit intense for the woman. Therefore, she should support herself by placing her hands on his chest, rib cage or thighs.

Considering that the woman is completely in charge in this position, she should begin by sliding up and down the shaft of his manhood by raising and lowering her lower body. The woman's up and down movements should be a variation of fast and shallow thrusts that only massage the tip of his member, then proceed to deep and gradual thrusts that cover the shaft of his penis entirely. The mind-blowing friction caused by the woman's movements will give the man the triple bonus of extraordinary sensations on his penis. In addition, to spice up the whole ordeal, the woman can arch her back or lean forward to create room for the man to fondle.

Why is it effective?

Just a couple of minutes into this sex position, a man and his partner will rapidly realize why this sex position has a very impressive climax capability for the man. A woman lingering in a suggestive or arousing squat on top of the man, instead of the normal straddling or sitting on him gives the woman the perfect conditions to tightly clench the man's sexual organ with her vagina. This sex position presents the woman with the easiest way to flex her PC muscles around the man's glans area of the penis. This can, in turn, trigger a powerful orgasmic reaction. This erotic sex position equally gives the woman enough room to take control of depth and pace of thrusts which in turn strips the man of control over the entire sex experience hence he barely has control of his climax because the woman's variation of shallow and deep movement tease the penis. A woman squatting above the man gives her the ability to exploit the entire shaft of the penis and this will consequently boost the intensity of the man's pleasure.

The sensual sidewinder

How to do it

Here, the man should be facing the woman as they both lie down on their sides. The man should then raise the woman's leg to create space for his Penetration. The woman's leg should be firmly placed on top of that of the man in such a way that it will not move too much when the man starts thrusting. It is also important to ensure that both the man's and lady's feet are placed against a hard immobile surface like a wall. This is particularly important for the man because it provides him with the support he needs to thrust in the way he sees fit The tension in the man's legs as he thrusts builds up the pressure to reach climax.

The woman's thighs should be loosely clasped together in a manner that envelops the man's penis. The woman's thighs tightly clasp the man's penis in a manner that results into some sort of friction hence the man reaches climax in the long run. The man can also use the free hand to fondle and caress the woman as he initiates kisses and eye contact

Why is it effective?

The sensual sidewinder supports the lazy and leisurely speed that eventually result in intense orgasmic reactions. Taking the entire process slowly and steadily will definitely win the climax trophy because orgasmic reactions that are a result of lengthy and gradual buildups are usually much more intense than those that are achieved by intense and fast stimulation. Taking time to savour every sensation enables you to experience an elevated degree of pleasure. If you accelerate from zero to one hundred very quickly, you will be "dropped off" faster, however, if you build up your momentum from zero to twenty, fifty and so on your engine will be very hot and steamy by the time you get to one hundred. In addition, this side-by-side position cultivates intimacy that can get lost in vigorous sexual activities. The closeness, eye contact and kisses will completely arouse a man and in the long run, his orgasmic reactions will be very intense.

.

The mystic missionary

How to do it

The man should penetrate the woman as she lies on her back with her legs spread apart. As soon as the man gets inside, he should bring the woman's legs together and then proceed to place his ankles around the woman's calves and slightly raise his body with a subtle arch on his back. He will create a picture of something that looks more or less like a frog but the sensations and pleasure that come with it will make him feel like a king. The woman closing her legs creates a strained entry for the man and consequently more and more glans stimulation

Why is it effective?

The mystic missionary position is a slightly improvised form of the normal missionary position. It a perfect recipe for a man's maximum pleasure and eventual orgasm because it makes his penis very firm and also gives some intense stimulation to his glans. This is because the man's and woman's stay locked together during the entire sexual activity because the sensations and heat that result from this are very pleasurable. Most importantly, the position is important to the man because it results in some type of muscle contraction that can be mind-blowing. It is a position that does not require too much energy, however, the movements involved put the man's body in movements that are more pleasure enhancing as opposed to the normal missionary position because it gives the man more room for squeezing and consequently build up his arousal.

CoItal alignment

How to do it

Kick it off in the traditional missionary style with the woman lying on her back and the man on top of the woman, strategically positioned in between her legs. The should then pull his upper body forward towards the woman's head so that his pelvic region is a little bit high up on the woman's body as opposed to how it happens in the normal missionary position. Rather than thrusting in and out, the man should strive to grind against the woman's pelvic area.

Why is it effective?

In spite of the fact the name sounds a little bit clinical, this is a very great position for any man who is seeking to boost his sexual pleasures and eventual orgasms. It creates more intimacy because the man can establish and maintains eye contact with the woman. He might also spice up the whole process by incorporating kisses on the lips and other erogenous zones of the woman like the neck. This builds intimacy that is an important recipe for a man's bid to experience more sexual pleasure. In addition, the positioning of the man's mid-section implies that his member is deep inside the walls of the vagina. This deep penetration means that the tip of his penis is constantly rubbing on the deeply rooted walls of the vagina, thus creating a sensation that is extremely pleasurable. In addition to the fact that is stress-free and intimate, it is easier for the man to shift from this position to missionary position and other positions thereafter. This changes in position ensure that various regions of the man's penis are stimulated hence the pleasure is much more intense because it is not concentrated in one place.

The cowgirl

How to do it

In this case, the man lies on his back and then the woman comes on top of the man with her legs placed on either side of the man's torso. After the penis penetrates the vagina, the woman proceeds to rock her body back and forth. It is important to note that the bat and forth movements are way more effective than trying to bounce up and down. The woman can also opt to grind her pelvic region in slow motion as if she is trying to write the letters of the alphabet with her waist.

Why is it effective?

In as much as men are obsessed with a depth of Penetrating a woman, they equally desire the pleasure that comes about due to anticipation. This is where teasing works wonders. I'm this position, in as much as the woman is in charge of pleasing herself and teasing the man, the man has the ability to thrust as slow or as fast as he can from below by pulling her closer to his chest. There are also numerous variations of fun that can be executed in this position making it extremely versatile hence the man has the ability to experience a variety of pleasurable feelings from the various variations that are applicable to this position. In addition, the man is in a position to maintain eye contact with the woman for purposes of intimacy and his hands are also free to explore the woman's body, caressing and fondling her erogenous zones.

Variations.

The woman can turn away and face the man's feet with her legs still straddled on either side of the man's torso. This is usually referred to as the reverse cowgirl. This is also pleasurable to the man in the sense that he is able to fondle and caress other desirable parts of the woman's body like the buttocks, waist or back. It gives the man a pleasing view.

The doggy style

How to do it

Here, the woman gets on her hands and knees. The man then kneels behind her in a position that he can easily penetrate the woman. The man can hold onto the woman's hips or waist and thrust at a pace that he sees fit. The woman has the option of staying still or bumping her hips back against the man.

Why is it effective?

The doggy style gives the man a better view of the action and his pleasure comes from giving the woman pleasure. I'm addition, I'm this position, the man takes control of the depth and pace of Penetration. Being in control gives him the authority to thrust in ways that are pleasurable to him, irrespective of whether it involves deep or shallow thrusts.

In this position, the man's hands are also free to explore the parts of the woman's body that he desires to touch. He can caress the woman's breasts, back or even take things a notch higher by teasing her clitoris.

Variations

In this position, the woman can change the angle in which the man is penetrating by going down on her elbows. The man can also opt to get more balance by getting out of bed and standing on the floor as the woman stands on all fours on the bed. Nonetheless, the bed has to be in such a way that the man does not struggle to thrust or penetrate. A man thrusts are more intense when he is standing on his feet.

The woman could also go down with the stomach first and then the man slightly lies on top of her and thrusts away.

Lap dance

In this position, the woman is treating the man top something a little bit more special. Here, the man sits down upright on a chair and then the woman slowly approaches him and straddles him. All that a man has to do here is sit back and enjoy the pleasure of being teased. You could also use his hands to fondle and caress the woman.

Scissor missionary

It starts off as the ordinary mission position but the woman goes ahead to put one of her legs on top of the man's shoulder as she holds the other leg onto the bed.
It is pleasurable to men in the sense that it limits the partner's movement from the action, therefore, a man can feel the pleasure of the women being in control of the woman. He becomes the dominant

Dragonfly

This sex position is especially good for men who are in love with penetration visuals. It gives him a clear view of every aspect of the sexual activity as well as the features of the woman like the breasts and clitoris.

In this position, the man sits with his legs stretched out as he supports his weight with his hands firmly placed behind him on the ground or bed. The woman then sits facing the man with one or both of his kegs placed on the man' s shoulder.

Chapter 8: Positions Suitable for Oral Sex Performed On Him

Oral sex can be instrumental in improving an individual's or a couple's sex life. In the case of women, oral sex prior to intercourse helps in loosening the vaginal muscles as well as increasing lubrication whereas, for men, it helps in having stronger erections by increasing the flow of blood to the penis. However, finding the oral sex position that works for you is a game of trial and error. In this chapter, we take a look at some oral sex positions that you can try on your man.

The kneeling oral sex position

The kneeling oral sex position is considered as the standard oral sex position for administering oral sex to a man. To perform the kneeling oral sex position on your man, he as to be in a position where he is facing you after which you go ahead and get on to your knees as your man maintains his position standing upright. On your knees, your head will be pretty much in line with his pelvic region, thus making it easier to administer the oral sex.

.How to do it

Just from the name, you can already create a vivid picture of what it is. Basically, the man stands in an almost upright posture and then the woman shows submission by kneeling on the ground and pleasuring him.

Another crucial point is that if the partners have agreed on it, he can make use of his hand to hold the back the woman's head and consequently thrust her head gently towards his groin. These thrusts might get intense when he is overwhelmed by the sensation of the woman's tongue and lips working on his member. Take that not everybody likes the thrusting idea, therefore make sure that you ask them whether they are comfortable with you doing that.

The man could also use the hand placed behind his partner's head to gently pull her closer as she takes in the man's manhood into the mouth. These slow and gentle thrusts help the man to determine the depth and speed in which the manhood goes in and out of the mouth.

In case the woman has long hair that flows all the way to her face, he could make use of the free hand to hold her hair for her to prevent them from being an obstruction to the process of oral sex. In addition, if the hair keeps on bothering her, her mind might wander off the oral sex so that she could concentrate on the hair.

Why you should love the kneeling oral sex position?

As we mentioned earlier, a lot of people consider the kneeling oral sex position as the standard oral sex position whereas in some instances, others consider it boring. Nonetheless, over the years, it has maintained its title the supreme oral sex position because it has numerous variations to it and you do not have to necessarily be flexible to execute it.

Another advantage is that getting into a Kneeling position is something that can be done almost instantly. Therefore, it comes in handy in cases where you and your partner get overwhelmed with the heat of the moment. All you have to do is kneel and get down to business.

Taking into consideration that the oral sex position can be carried out on a number of places like the couch, the bed, and on a chair, you and your partner are definitely spoilt for choice. Therefore, you have to discuss with him so that you carry out a little bit of an experiment to figure out what works for both of you.

This type of oral sex position is great because it gives the woman enough room to move back and forth as well as up and down as she administers the oral sex

Additional tips on the kneeling oral sex position

1. Make sure that you incorporate a lot of eye contact to ameliorate the intimacy and pleasure of oral sex.

2. Ensure that your knees are protected-In some cases the ground on which you are kneeling might be rough and you might end up getting bruises or even cuts. Therefore, consider using pillows or any other comfortable materials.

3. Where should you do it? – Just like normal sexual intercourse, the best place to give your man oral sex is in the bedroom. However, try to be adventurous or creative and try new places like the bathroom or the living room.

4. Squatting or kneeling? - In some instances, you might be in situations where you do not feel like kneeling on the hard floor. Squatting can be a great replacement for this.

5. Reach around- When you are on your knees, do not just kneel, there are a number of things you could do to spice up the whole thing. For example, you could use your hand to caress and fondle him to give him maximum pleasure.

Boss' Chair oral sex position

This oral sex position derives its name from the simple reason that your man will feel special because he is comfortably seated as you submissively kneel to please him. Therefore, it is an oral sex position where your man sits comfortably and in a relaxed posture as you administer oral sex on him.

How to do it

Make sure. that your man sits somewhere he feels comfortable and relaxed. He should sit in such a way that the spreads his legs leaving enough space in between the legs where his you can fit comfortably. The woman can then move into space between his legs and get down to businesses of pleasing him.

You might be forced to support your arms by placing them on the man's laps. You can choose to either squat or kneel depending on what works for boss chair

When to use the boss' chair oral sex position

If your man is in the bedroom with you, it is very easy to try this position, particularly if he is seated in the same way he sits on the couch, with his feet dangling slightly above the floor or on the floor. Another appropriate place to administer oral sex using the boss chair position would be in the living room area watching TV or when he is on the computer doing something.

Try to be as inconspicuous as possible. Do not openly show him that you intend to administer oral sex because ambushes will definitely yield more results. For instance, if he is seated like a "boss" on the couch watching TV with his legs widespread, just walk up to him and get into position and go-ahead to give him oral sex. It will catch him off-guard and he will like it.

Extra tips for the Boss Chair Oral Sex Position

1. Role-play-A very excellent way to catapult the Boss' chair position to a completely new level would be by bringing up an element of role-playing or fantasy. For instance, you could start off by putting on a sexy dress so that you look like a model and then go over to where he is and play that fantasy role as you administer oral sex to him.

2. A surprise at half time-Whenever you and your man are having alone time at home and you are probably watching your favourite team play on TV, be patient until the half time period and then go into the bedroom and change into something he will find hard to resist. Perhaps lingerie, and then go back to where he is and make sure you do not say a word, just get into the boss 'chair position and get into action right away. It is a guarantee that your man will feel extremely pleasured.

3. Tie down-If you are of the idea of being a little bit dominant and you are sure he is okay with it, you could try to tie his hands and legs onto the chair before administering the oral sex.

Regular Oral Sex Position

The regular oral sex position is arguably the only oral sex technique that majority of girls employ on their men during sex in the bedroom.

How to go about The Regular oral sex Position
The regular oral sex position is probably one of the easiest technique of administering oral sex. Here, the man has to lie on his back on the bed or any other comfortable surface with his legs spread widely. Thereafter, you have to lie down on either side of your man and make sure that your head is positioned close to his pelvic region. Whenever you are comfortable and ready, all that you have to do is get down to business.

Extra tips on how to do the regular oral sex position

1. Switch off the lights- If you have ever administered oral sex before, then you must have realized that sometimes you might feel anxious or even nervous. The best way to solve this problem and do away with the nervousness would be to switch off the lights before going down to give him oral sex. If the first option does not work for you, the second option would be to administer the oral sex underneath the beddings. It is normal for some people to act shy whenever they give their man oral sex because they know the man is looking at them, or maybe they have the fear that they are not doing it the right way whereas others are simply shy. If you match any of the descriptions above, try out the solutions mentioned above. They might be a game-changer for

you.

2. Incorporate your hands-Whenever you go down on your man for quite some time, you might find out that jaw and mouthy start to feel fatigued. The best way to give the jaws and mouth a break as you continue satisfying your man would be by using your hands as a substitute for the mouth.

3. Foreplay- Just like intercourse, for oral sex also to be pleasurable, you have to prepare your man psychologically Set the mood before getting down to business. You have to make a smooth transition from the foreplay to going down on him. You can begin by straddling him, caressing him, kissing him from his lips followed by his neck, then chest and stomach so that by the team you get to the crotch he will be extremely ready for the oral sex.

4. Caressing the stomach-When you are down to the business of giving him oral sex, make an attempt to caress his stomach or chest. Doing this cultivates so much intimacy in comparison to performing oral sex alone.

5. Tie your hair or request that he holds it for you- If your hair is long and you have a feeling that it will get into your way, make an effort to tie it before the auction begins. However, or if you get caught up in the moment, you can simply ask him to hold it for you.

Cinema Oral Sex Position

The cinema oral sex position is where both the man and the woman are sitting next to each other, side-by-side just the same way they sit in cinemas. In this position, all you have to do is lean over, unzip your man's fly and get down to business. As you do so. your man remains seated the same way he was seated.

It is important to note that the Cinema Oral Sex Position does not have to be necessarily performed in a cinema. As long as you are seated side-by-side in a comfortable place, you can perform this position.

Take everything slow

If you have never performed oral sex before, I am sure you are curious and you really want to try it out. However, it is important to come to the realization that most men appreciate if you systematically build-up to the main event. Therefore, rather than just jumping onto your man's zip, it would be better if you started off gradually.

To begin with, you could caress him using your hands with a special focus on his testicles and penis. Do it gently for some time in a way that will arouse him. Thereafter reach for his pants and gently but steadily tease his penis and testicles. This should go on for a few minutes so that the sexual urge in him keeps growing. After this, you can now take the big step and go-ahead to perform oral sex.

Extra Tips for Cinema Oral Sex Position

1. Give your man some control- The greatest way to make that moment worthwhile, particularly if you are the kind of woman that likes a man who is always in control, give him the mantle of controlling the depth as well as the pace. He can do this by placing his hand at the back of your head so that he controls the back and forth movements. However, if you are not for the idea, then you tell him that you do not like it that way.

2. Make use of your hands –The cinema oral sex position does not require you to use your hand to support yourself. Therefore, this means that you can use it to massage his testicles and stroke his penis in turns.

The Thigh Pillow Position

This oral sex position is ideal for those lazy days because it is relaxed more than the other positions like the cinema position.

How the Thigh Pillow Oral Sex Position is Performed
Performing this oral sex position on your man requires that you make use of his thigh as a pillow. Here, your man has to first position himself properly by lying on his side, then he should place his legs in such a way that leg that is on the mattress is in front whereas the other leg is stretched out at the back. He should also make sure that the leg at the back stays exactly where it is. Now, move in and take up your position by laying down on your side and then proceed to place your head on the thigh of the leg that is in front. In this position, your

head will be directly linked with your crotch, therefore, all you have to do is give him oral sex.

Additional Tips for the Thigh Pillow Oral Sex Position

1. You can wrap around-You can opt to be more comfortable by holding by firmly holding your man's other thigh or even his waist to draw him closer to you.
2. The thigh pillow position enables you to lie down in opposite directions with your man, where your head is where his feet are and vice versa. This position can allow you to perform oral sex on your man easily. All you have to do is pull or push yourself to a position where your head is lined up with his pelvic region. On the other end, your man could also return the favour by performing oral sex on you as well.
3. Explore Other Places other than the Bedroom- Something else that is fascinating about the thigh pillow position is that you do not have to necessarily do it in bed. Be creative and try other options like performing it on a large couch or a floor that has been carpeted.

Chapter 9: Five Positions Suitable for Oral Sex Practiced on Her

Oral sex is entirely different from other types of intimacies. It will not be possible for her to get pregnant when you have oral sex since it is safer. Many men are never ready to give their partners the satisfaction that they need and they are forced to do oral sex. When you practice oral sex with time, it can help make your sex life varied. You will be in a position to understand your partner well and more about what they like in sex and what they do not like. You will know more about how they feel and what they desire. You need to be confident when you are practicing this and make sure that your partner is satisfied as well. When you trust each other, you will find it enjoyable.

Oral sex may get monotonous with time, and you need to find new ideas to use on her so that you will not get bored. When you want to play oral sex, you have to be aware of the tie as well as place, that is something that you should not ignore since it will affect the quality of the oral sex. There are times when she will feel like she can no longer keep silent, and she needs to scream. Make sure that you are not in a place that you will distract people since this is a two people affair and not the entire world. Work towards the same goal, to make your partner feel that there is someone who cares about them. Make them know that you have a special feeling towards her. Know that you can sex for a different purpose. Know the main goal so that you will stick to that. Make use of your hands as well as tongue to explore the treasure that she posses so that you can spice up the oral sex.

It is not wrong to keep changing the positions so that you will know that best fits for you. Changing the styles from time to time will make a significant difference when you come to the foreplay. When you practice the new approaches, you never know where it will head to on that particular night. It will not only be right for you but also her if she cannot get to orgasm from the penetration sex. You can either do foreplay as the main event or just for fun. Some of the oral sex positions will go in favour of men. Some will work best when you on a woman. Find out more about them.

However, there are different oral sex styles that you can try on her, and they will work out. They include and not limited to;

The Shark Fin

The shark fin will not be possible when you want to pull off the underwater. Let her lie back on a towel or a cloth, and place their hips on the tub edge. Spread her legs and make sure that the feet dangle in the water. Use your mouth to work on her and make sure she will appreciate what you will do no her. When doing this, you will create a good as well as a strong bond between both of you. If you notice that your partner is comfortable with the position they are in, they can maintain that for a more extended period. If they are not healthy, you can consider changing the style to a more comfortable one. Make sure it will be a win-win for both of you. Work on your partner until they are satisfied since you are doing that for fun. It should be enjoyable, and both of you should enjoy the play. When you are out for any sex, you must maintain hygiene. When she is clean, you will not find it hard to use your tongue to shift her in another world. Change the position once you know that she is tired since you do not want to make her feel exhausted before you work on them appropriately.

The Butterball

It is an excellent position for cunnilingus as well as a rim job. You can even decide to get a shower with her so that you can prepare her from the word go. Make her lie back, and her knees should bend towards their chest. The position will not only be sweet for her, but it will help you to have access to her breast as well as her clitoris. She will as well have access to your butt, penis as well as testicles. That is a perfect recipe for satisfaction, and that will help both of you to be stimulating for fun. When that happens, you will have reached the aim of your play which is satisfaction and enjoyment. If you think that a barrier will work for you rimming and you do not have a dental handy, the best thing for you is to get hold of some plastic wrap and use it instead. You need to be clean for each other when you decide to go the butterball oral sex. First, take a shower, and you can do it together to make sure that the oral sex will be sweeter. The more you spend a lot of time in the intimacy temperature, the more it will be calm when you get into the real action. Know that this sex position will be significantly influenced by any work that you will do to shut down your partner. If something is bothering you, you will have wicked pleasure. When you insert the face in her honey pot, you can make her play along with your penis, and if possible, she can give you some blow job. It is an excellent position if you need her to do some blow job.

All Hail the Queen

It is one way of saying that she should sit on your face. You need to lie on your back so that she can straddle your face and she will kneel in front of you. It does not mean that she sits on your face, but it can be so if you need her to smother you. The style will give her thighs a light workout as she will be trying to hover a few inches above your head. It is not painful, and she will find pressure all along. You too will enjoy working on her. If you want her to sit on your face, that will mean that you want a killer vagina. The position will be an advantage to you since you will be in a place to hold her butt as well as hips. And bearing in mind, no one does not like to touch the butt, or their butt touched. Your girl will get to the orgasmic throne in a moment, and she will like it. Be ready to worship the girl when the time comes, and she will take commands of the erotic powers as well as control over the sensation. You can try to make her aroused by playing with her breasts. You can tease her with the vibrating breast teaser that will make her feel the pleasure. It is a sweet moment and a one to remember. Enjoy each other and be free to make the oral sex graduate to something else. In cases where it gets to something else, that will be the sweetest sex ever since you have had excellent foreplay. Do it until she surrenders and be sure that she has had all the pleasure in the world. The breast teaser will send a charge directly to her breasts and will send all, the heat in her whole body. It will be a good time for her to yell what she feels for you. Do it until she is satisfied. The position will help out both of you in a dominant role. When your head is between her thighs, you can start working on making her feel like a queen. Treat that girl like a queen and make sure that she is in that position that she feels comfortable. When she is relaxed, you will give her the best, and she will respond refreshingly. Let your girl know that she should not place all her weight on your face. That will make you inactive, and it will mean you will not do an excellent job on her. Make sure that you have breathing space so that you will not suffocate. You can support her with your hands when she gets tired, and you can help with your hands under the thighs. You girl will feel special when you use this position, and that means that you get a live crown on your head. That is just so amazing.

The Cliffhanger

Let her sit on the end of your bed, and her booty should be at the very end. You need to make sure that her legs dangle off the end. You will kneel in front of her so that you can make confident that your face will be in an angle that is towards the vagina. That will allow you to get the clitoris in the right corner, and you will not struggle to stimulate her. When you do that, you will get into a world of you own in a flash of a second. Your hands will be free to move in the direction they want and to touch all her body in the way it pleases you. You can tease her favourite zones, and you can even opt to double down on her vagina. You will reach the climax in a moment, and you cannot deny that it is an excellent style. When she is on this style, you can play around with her nipples, and that will give that both of you double pleasure. It can as well be called bon appétit oral sex position where you will put your head in between her thighs. You can make her pull her legs apart in a v shape. She can close ankles around your neck, and you will find more pleasure. When she gets tired, or she is no longer comfortable with the position, she can lie down while you go down to work on her.

Sofa King Good

Make your partner lie on the couch and the back and the head on the seat. Be sure that their legs draped. It is your turn now to play your part and make them feel appreciated. Kneel over her face, and you face the back of the couch. The next thing you need to do is bend over and do the necessary. Doing it on the sofa will make you relax than doing in bed, and you will find it enjoyable. You will find pleasure both you and your partner since it is a cool thing to do. It is a good chance for you to give as well as receive the game at the same time. It can be acrobatics in one way or the other. You can stabilize your girl using your legs, and that will be a bit relaxing.

The sofa king good oral sex position will derive double pleasure. For both, you and your partner will feel the sweetness that is in the play. No one will be left unsatisfied, and both of you will love the idea. Anytime that you think your partner needs this style of sex, they will not hesitate to give you. That is because it has a fulfilling experience that you would like to try out any time that you have a chance to. Make sure that your girl is not hurting. The best place to do this oral sex is on the couch. It will give you more pleasure than doing it in bed. The sofa has a unique way to make her stay in the angle that you want and the one that you will a have access to all she is. Make it sweet for her that she will wish to reciprocate it to you. That will be a way to show you that they appreciate what you are doing on them. When they decide to return, it can be smoothing better like making you penetrate in her honey pot. The sex will be just the best since you have presided it with fantastic foreplay. Do not make her leave the couch if she has not reached orgasm and you as well need to cum so that you will feel satisfied.

The sweetest oral sex positions are intimate, sensual as well as dynamic, and that is what will make the play more pleasurable. The skills, as well as experience that your partner will use to make the game huge, is a significant factor that will decide the pleasure that you will have. It will as well determine whether you will get to orgasm. When your girl tells you what to do, it is good that you do it because that will make her feel right. Communicate with her so that she can be open and tell you what she wants you to do. The position that both you and your girl will enjoy is the best for you. Be clear and do not fail to tell your partner what you feel and whether the position is hurting or bringing more pleasure. When they do you a favour, do not forget to return it. It the guy gives you a tasty treat, you as his lady should treat him as well. Appreciate one another when it comes to this fantastic play, and it will be more enjoyable.

Oral sex is a great recipe to spice up your union. You will have fantastic sex, and you need to know that both the parties in the receiving and the giving side should be active. Do not forget that any kind f sex is necessary for your relationship. Do not restrict the definition of sex as just penetration; it can be oral as well. The oral sex will make your relationship to be healthy as well as a balanced diet. At times, penetration is less intimate when you compare with oral sex. For both of you to enjoy, you need to be creative. Find out the best sex position, and you will get to the pleasure that you are looking. When you do it, and you expose you body parts in the air, the sweeter and better it will be. Be spontaneous, and that will make the other partner enjoy even though they did not want it. It is upon you to make it as enjoyable as it can. If you find it shy to do when there is light, switch them off so that you will forget about everything and maintain your focus.

Chapter 10: Five Positions Suitable for Anal Sex in Which She Finds More Pleasure and Less Discomfort

In some time back, anal sex was a taboo, but as days go by, couples are adding it in their sex life. It was an experience that was felt once n a while, and it was not universal. When women did it, they did it for the sake of their parents but not because they were enjoying what they were doing. Couples are adopting anal sex as time goes on, and they find pleasure in it. It is getting in the mainstream with time. A lot of women are talking about it everywhere and the fun they see when they do the anal sex. The nerves, as well as the pleasure points that are around and inside the anus, will make you have the sweetest sex ever.

When you do anal sex, you are giving the body time to relax as well as a warm-up. You need to go step by step so that you will avoid the pain that can come from the sex and you will not find t comfortable. You may not be sure of your partner's health status, and you have to take care of yourself. There are no exceptions, and you are supposed to use protection, preferably a condom.

When you are a beginner or even you are used to the anal sex, you can consider trying one of these styles. They are comfortable, fun as well as intimate. They include and not limited to;

Backside Doggy Position

Any time that you think of doing anal sex, your mind will rush to the doggy style. It is normal, and you do not need to understand the reason behind. You will be in a position to penetrate quickly, and you will have control over your girl. The place will be a perfect angle of penetration, and you will derive more pleasure. First, you need to make sure that she is on her fours. You are the next person to position yourself, and you need to kneel behind her and place your hands n her hips. Once you are sure that your girl is ready to have it from you, do the necessary. Place the tip of your penis on her entry point. Make her shift her hips if it is essential, backward, and forward so that she can have the control of the depth as well as rhythm. Aim to go deeper in her, and you will find pleasure. It is likely that when you go deeper in her, you will hit her A-spot. The spot is highly sensitive as well as pleasurable. When you can stimulate this spot, they will likely have an anal orgasm.

For you to make sure that both of you are having maximum pleasure, change your body angles from time to time. Let her start on her fours, and you will know how it feels, and you decide whether you will change or you first enjoy for some time and then change. Make her lower her chest on the bed and know how it feels. Take care of your partner, making sure that they will not tire before you reach the maximum point. You can make use of your fingers as well as hands so that you can trigger more urge to play the game. The more urgent the both of you will feel, the higher the chances that you will enjoy. Sweet anal sex will be as a result of the both of you knowing what will trigger you and work that out.

Cowgirl Anal

It is anal sex, whereas the girl will be on top of you when you try to make your pennies penetrate in her. Your girl will recline facing up and the knees on either side of you. That will mean that her legs will be apart while she is on top of you. You can choose to start the game, or she can begin. That will depend on whatever you will agree. She will lower her booty in slow motion onto your penis, and she will adjust until the moment she feels you are. She will find the best position until she will feel comfortable. Give a chance to drive you, and you as well enjoy the pleasure. Let her grind, rock as well as roll her hips until the time that she will find a rhythm that both of you will enjoy. Do not just stay r-there to feel the pleasure. Sex is a two way, and you need to make your partner enjoy the same way you are doing. If they are not enjoying, then that is not sex, but it is likely to be rape. You can touch her clit as a way to make her feel stimulated, and she will make it amazing for you. The position will stimulate her G-spot, and she will reach orgasm in no time. As a way to boost her, you can decide to use a vibrator against her clitoris, and you can add other approaches that will stimulate so that you can reach to a wild pleasure.

Butt Lifted Missionary

The position is among one of the intimate anal sex. You will enjoy it when you decide to use a pillow to lift her hips. It is enjoyable, and you will not regret thinking about it. It is a great idea to play it, and it will create a strong bond between you and her. When she lay n her back, put a pillow under her hips and another one under her head. You have to support your weight with your hands and enter her slowly. Make sure that she will feel it when you enter her and if possible, make her yell a little. The yelling should not be because of pain, but pleasure, she is feeling when you are sliding inside her. She can opt to help you do it better by placing her hands on your hips. When she does this, you will be in a position to access the tempo that will make her feel as if she is in another world. The sweetness of that spot will make her find the pleasure that she wants.

Make her get hold of the back of her knees and take them closer to her chest. That will make you slip in quickly, and you will go deeper in a way that she will like it. There is nothing that she will enjoy when you dig deep in her. The deeper you will go, the likely hood that she will feel more pleasure. Once you are sure that she finds a rhythm that makes her feel good, you can direct her to stimulate her clit using her fingers or a vibrator. Be in control and make sure you pay attention to any form of non-verbal communication. It can be hard for her to talk when she is feeling you penetrate inside her like never before. When she is not able to utter any word, that is the time you know that she has gone in the pleasure. Respond to her touches or signals that she will give you to either go slowly or make it quicker. That will make both of you find comfort in the anal sex, and you will enjoy each other. Your girl will like it sometime when you get deeper and deeper in her, that is when you feel that she is not the same innocent girl anymore and she is enjoying the sexing. Make it feel as sweet as you can, and she will not deny you it any other time that you will need her. She will be longing for that time that you will say of anal sex, and she will ready to receive it from you.

Backdoor Side-By-Side

If you are a beginner of anal sex, this is a good position for you to start. It will introduce you to the rest of the anal sex styles. It is comfortable and will make her anal muscles to relax as she waits for you to work on her. Let her lie on her sides and the curl around her in a spoon style. As she is laying little spoon, get in her slowly by slowly and inch by inch. You are the one who needs to control her in the best way to put it inside her. If you want to dig deeper in her, you can ask her to back up her butt, and you will find it easy as well as faster to go deeper in the honey pot.

Careless her as you shower her with kisses will make it more enjoyable. Kiss her ears and neck as you feel her adjust till she perceives you. That will make your game intimate, and you will enjoy each other. It is the best feeling that you will ever have. As a beginner, you will love the anal sex more, and you will always look forward to the moment she will give it to you once more. She will reach orgasm, and you will enjoy calming inside her. The intimacy will come by the fact that you can get hold of her clit and play with it as you feel the warmth inside her.

On Bended Knee

The position will need her to lie on her side, and you will be snuggled up behind your girl. Let her draw her top knee towards her chest and make sure that her bottom led extended. Now your chance is here to have a taste of her. Find you way slowly inside your girl as she will be holding her butt wide open so that you can find your way with ease. Know that you are the one who is in charge of how deep you will go and the speed in which you will ride her. Change the angle of their knee to the position that you desire so that you can stimulate the senses, and she will have it all. The place is comfortable for you to personalize, and that makes it the favourite. There are many varieties, and you can change her in the way that pleases you and the one that you feel you can enjoy the juicy her. You can go to the depth that you think will make her scream of how sweet you are. You are free to touch any part of her body to create more intimacy since your hands will not be supporting anything. Hold her tight and make sure that she gets the best out of the game.

You cannot run up on your partner any time that you need to pay anal sex. Prepare her for some few hours that in a moment you will have a taste of her. That will make it sweeter since she will be ready to receive the entire you. Anal sex will give you pleasure to the extent that you will want to play it all the time. When you go anal sex for some time, you will realize that her sphincter will relax and it will get more enjoyable with time.

Do not stick to one position, but you have to try out other posts. Experiment with shallow as well as short strokes and know how it feels. You can try the deep and long penetrations to see the one that both of you will prefer. Alternate between the two and you will establish the exact one that you will find more pleasure. Do it in different angles and know the one that will work best for you. Add a little dominance as well as submission play so that you will have great sex. You can choose to dominate, or your girl does, and you will have the hottest sex ever.

You need to take your time together with your partner so that you can talk about your sex life. Do not talk about it indirectly but immediately address things, and it is healthy. It is good to give your partner some feedback on how the game was after the entire layer is over. Tell them the exact thing that they do when in the game which does not please you. Make sure that they give you the feedback as well.

Chapter 11: Toys: When to Use Them and How

In some years back, the use of sex toys was taboo. However, the popularity of these toys, as well as their usage in marriage, have significantly changed. Nowadays, the taboos surrounding vibrators, as well as other sex toys, are dissolving with time. People who used to condemn the use of these toys publicly are even suing them to satisfy their sexual drive. Also, the incidence of infections, as well as the emergence of conditions that have no cure, such as HIV, has increased the rate at which people are avoiding real sex. The art of unfaithfulness in marriage has also been the primary cause of the current use of sex toys. In other words, people are following the taboo that if you buy a sex toy unless you give it to someone which is a rare case, it will never cheat on you. However, in real marriages, men and women are sleeping with other people other than their real partners. There are a lot of injustices happening in marriages. Men and women are killing each other due to jealousy. Others are signing in divorces due to the art of not being sexually satisfied marriage. There are other women who after being betrayed by their partners; they resolve never to love a man again. After making such a resolution, sexual desires doesn't end.

In most cases, they are forced to look for alternatives or rather other ways of satisfying their sexual urge. In most cases, the best option for many of them remains to the use of sex toys. Thus, it is essential to understand when to use sex toys and how to use them as well.

Changing the Mind-set

The art of enhancing sexual pressure undoubtedly increases the enjoyment therein. It is worth noting that the best sexual entertainment or enhancement is created in the minds. In other words, people who enjoy their marriage to the fullest or engage in satisfactory sexual behaviours start it in their mind. In the same way, people who cherish the use of these toys can site the art of changing their mindset being the route or rather the primary aspect that causes them to enjoy ti their fullest. Thus, as you explore the use of these toys, you need to adjust your minds and avoid the art of feeling guilty. It will make you hate sex for-ever. However, if you practice it intending to meet your sexual urge, you will do it correctly and reach orgasm with ease. You will be able to appreciate the creativity in you as well as be in an excellent position to explore the area that works best for you. It is also an excellent time to investigate your body and mark some of the places that drive you crazy about touching. Thus, you need to change your mindset and focus on meeting your sexual urge. You need to appreciate the art of having all these minds as well as the self-will of doing all these. The art is linked to the fact that there are individuals who don't have the ability as well as the feelings you might be having. Change your mindset and work on ensuring that you reach the highest climax. Explore all the parts of your body and ensure that the toy is working in the best way possible. Create some space on you to ensure that you are not disturbing anyone. It is worth noting that when using these toys, you aren't after Cumming or climaxing. However, you should aim at enjoying and feeling satisfied. Thus, you need to do is with a supper mindset that will allow you to stay for long without reaching orgasm, and when you climax, you will feel relieved. Thus, you need to adhere to a positive mindset.

Avoiding false Beliefs

If you want to enjoy the use of sex toys, you need to be categorical and avoid false beliefs. One of the most disturbing conclusions is that sex toys are used by partners who aren't able to satisfy their wives sexually. Others believe that owning or using a toy is a sign of breakage in marriage or lack of trust. However, the aspect depends on how you set your minds as well as the things you believe in. It is worth noting that what matters is the agreement you have with your partner. Also, the situation at hand determines the way one perceives everything.

If you believe in such false-hood, the chances are that you wont enjoy you wont enjoy. You will feel much guilty at the end, and you might even hate your partner. However, if you can agree and understand your partner, you will be able to enjoy and use it effectively. Others believe that the size of the toy or rather the penis matters. Some thus go for the large-sized toys for satisfaction. It is worth noting that what matter is whatever is done. In other words, you can have a small toy and put yourself in a good position and enjoy to the fullest rather than having a large doll that makes you feel uncomfortable. You also need to understand yourself well. In other words, know the things as well as the activities that quickly disturb you. You need to understand the places you go and feel more satisfied. Avoid such situations and create in your mind that you are after meeting an individual need that can be best achieved using a toy. Appreciate the toy you can afford and the feelings you have as well. You also need to understand the fact that you have the sexual drive and are willing to be satisfied. Make use all the time you have and the toys you can access and enjoy irrespective of the things people believe or say.

Appropriate way

There are cases when the male partner feels weak or fail to allow their partners to reach their climax. A lady may opt for the art of using such toys. In other cases, the partners may agree on the use of vibrators as well as other sex toys as they prepare for sex. Studies have revealed that there are men who can stay for long without Cumming after they use toys to make their loved one for sex. With a changed mind, the partners can enjoy the use of toys together. There are cases where your partner might be far, and you might be communicating with her or him on sex or rather how you long to have them in bed.

In most cases, such conversations end up in masturbation. In such situations, instead of using bare hands or rather miss the urge of climaxing, the best thing to use is a sex toy. In such a case, it causes one to lose their partners as they are the primary reason for using the toys. Ensure that the toy is of similar size with the penis of your partner. Also, it is good to use the position that satisfies you most when you are with your partner. If you are in a phone call, you can mourn and let them feel the enjoyment from far. The art will increase the way the two of you binds and may increase the urge of having sex with them.

Cleanliness

Your toys could be the source of infection if not used well. In most cases, when one climax or reach orgasm, one feels tired and quickly fall asleep. Thus, the toy may remain unclean for some time. The best thing to do is to consider the material of the gadget you are using. However, regardless of the content, make sure that the toys are always clean. You ca n also use disinfectants to ensure that the toy is safe from bacteria. It is still good to store them in a safe place and ensure that no dust reaches the site. At times, it is good to clean them before and after using them. The aspect ensures that no infections are spread in either way. There are cases where lesbians or rather homosexuals use similar toys due to sexual urge. In other words, there are times when the lesbians might be drawn much into satisfying their partners and end up forgetting the use of individual toys. In other cases, they may be forced to mix or use different toys as a means of finding more pressure. There are cases where some of these toys fall and collect some infections. However, due to the sexual urge and the desire to climax, one may forget even to wipe the toy off the dust. However, the best thing to do is to ensure that every time you are using the gadget, you have a disinfectant near you. In other words, before inserting the toy or instead of the vibrator you are using, wipe it, or clean it thoroughly. The aspect is critical in the sense that it helps one to minimize the rate of infections.

Understanding your Partner

In most cases, disputes, as well as fights in the marriage, occurs due to the art of misunderstanding. In most cases, the man or rather the woman may not be understanding the feelings of the manfully. In other words, the man may fail to know when and how to satisfy their partners to the fullest. In most cases, when men climax, they tend to assume that the ladies are well pleased, and they may not need more of the intimacy.

In most cases, it takes three to seven minutes for a man to climax after the first penetration. However, depending on how prepared the lady was, she might stay up to fifteen minutes.

The art indicates that when the man is climaxing, the lady is halfway and too far from reaching orgasm. The aspect shows that the man needs to have a second round of Cumming before the lady can climax. In such cases, if you can time and understand the time it takes for her to reach orgasm, you may opt using sex toys. In such situations, the lady will feel more appreciated as you aren't leaving them hanging. When a lady reaches orgasm, they feel valued and relax well. Most of them don't even have to climax two times for a single session. One climax is enough to satisfy the lady sexually. Thus, if you are tired after Cumming for the first time, you may use your hands or rather a toy that will help your partner to climax too. Thus, you need to understand how your partners behave when Cumming or when reaching orgasm. If during sex, you haven't reached the G-spot, ensure that you are extending your hand or instead of using the toy that will cause your partner to scream as she enjoys. Allow them to feel the presence of a partner who cares for their feelings as well. Create time for them and allow them to enjoy to the fullest.

Enabling Environment

It is worth noting that sex toys can drive someone crazy, and one may scream as they enjoy. In most cases, a gadget wont tire before you climax. It remains rigid and doing the same kind of job before and after climaxing. In other words, when a man climax, the size of their penis reduces. It requires more of caressing for it to regain its erectile position. However, a toy remains erect for its entire time. The aspect may drive a woman crazy, especially when Cumming. They may scream to the top of their voices and do all manner of things. The element indicates that you can't use a toy in any place. The aspect is linked to the fact that you may disturb other people's peace as you scream. It is thus useful to use the toys in a place far from others and or late at night when everyone is sincere in sleep. The aspect is critical in the sense that it allows one to be free at screaming or even rifting their legs high as they call anyone. Thus, next time you think of using toys, ensure that you create an enabling environment that will give you the art of being free and doing or saying anything.

Common Sex Toys

Bullet vibrator

When you are beginning to use sex toys, this is an excellent choice for you. It is sturdy as well as incredibly well-made. It is rechargeable, and you do not have to move around with batteries. It has the best stimulation ever, and you can choose to try it. It can never fail you and will give you the best satisfaction and will be fun to experience it. Your partner can use it during the play to stimulate your clit in preparation of great sex.

Silicone Dildo

It at all you are in love with dildos, this is a perfect choice for you. It will give you pleasure, and you can opt to add it in your collection. The satisfaction you will derive from using this sex toy will be one of a moment. It is fun to use, and it is likely to change its colour as the temperatures rise. It is affordable and will never frustrate you in any case. Try it out, and you will never regret it. Your partner can use it on you when you feel that you need more of it and he cannot work more on you.

Wand Vibrator

The wand dildos are very versatile, being for external use and for a direct stimulation of the clitoris, they are ideal for use during sex with the partner. The contemporary internal and external stimulation manages to give truly unique sensations. In couple sex it can be exploited in many positions, mainly in the missionary, with the woman resting on her back, holding the wand vibrator between you. In this position the weight of him will give the intensity to the vibration of the wand, and he will be able to manage it by removing weight, supporting himself with his arms. Another interesting position is the spoon, putting a few pillows under her belly. In this way the wand vibrator can be positioned from below, while the partner can penetrate from behind, making a nice sandwich for intense sensations.

www.ingramcontent.com/pod-product-compliance
Lightning Source LLC
Chambersburg PA
CBHW061704250726
48657CB00002B/525